Praise for *A Healthy Society, Updated and Expanded Edition*

"What do you get when an empathetic physician combines stories, concern for his community, and analysis? This special book. Ryan Meili goes from patient to society, and from social and political forces to the patient. If this book's insights were put into practice, we would get a healthy society indeed."

– MICHAEL MARMOT, director of UCL Institute of Health Equity and author of *The Health Gap*

"Meili speaks from experience, from the heart, and with passion for achieving social justice. His political insight in how to achieve prosperity for all citizens and society is creative and revolutionary."

– LOUISE SIMARD, former Saskatchewan minister of health and minister responsible for the status of women

"Understanding health means understanding society. Ryan Meili is a physician who understands both. This book is passionate, very readable, and gives the whole system a major push toward a better future."

– RICHARD WILKINSON, co-author of *The Spirit Level: Why More Equal Societies Almost Always Do Better*

"Physicians have traditionally sought to cure the ailing patient. Why are you not well? How can we make you well again? In this thoughtful and inspiring book, Ryan Meili takes this same approach to what ails us as a society. The perspective is holistic, novel, and necessary. If you want to know how we'll get to a better future for all, then you must read this book."

– YANN MARTEL, author of *The Life of Pi,* winner of the Man Booker Prize

"Dr. Meili's focus on health and its social determinants to drive social and political change is powerful. This book is written with clarity, centred on stories, and informed by years of experience as a family doctor and public policy reformer. Canadians would do well to heed its call to action to deepen our democracy through a focus on health."

– DANYAAL RAZA, chair of Canadian Doctors for Medicare

"It is a huge privilege to be allowed into people's individual stories as a family doctor, to come face to face with their most private fears and challenges. To do so while seeing the bigger picture, learning what can be generalized from each story, is the finest way to honour one's patients. The first edition of *A Healthy Society* brought upstream thinking to the mainstream, showing Canadians how a health lens could help us tackle our greatest challenges. The combination of story, evidence, and vision for the future in this latest edition is what we need to chart a path to a healthier Canada."

– DANIELLE MARTIN, author of *Better Now: Six Big Ideas to Improve Health Care for All Canadians*

"A vivid portrait of the adverse effects of current public policy directions upon the health of Canadians ... this volume is more timely than ever."

– DENNIS RAPHAEL, professor of health policy and management at York University and editor of *Social Determinants of Health: Canadian Perspectives*

"Collected in this book are stories most Canadians don't get to hear – stories that show that Canada can, and must, be a more compassionate country. *A Healthy Society* should be required reading for those tasked with crafting policy in this country, those pushing for a more caring Canada, and those interested in evidence-based decision-making."

– MAX FINEDAY, executive director of Canadian Roots Exchange

Praise for the First Edition

"We know it in our hearts: poor health is intimately linked to poverty, abuse, and lack of social services. Yet in all these areas, Canada is marching steadily backward. In *A Healthy Society*, Ryan Meili, a practising doctor who knows this first hand, sounds a clarion call to all Canadians. We will not have a healthy society until we put social justice and universal social security for all back at the top of our political agenda."

    — MAUDE BARLOW, honorary chairperson, Council of Canadians

"Dr. Meili makes a powerful argument: better health is a central narrative of our lives, our society, and our democratic institutions; so what's stopping us from walking the talk? A doctor's analytic eye diagnoses the problem: too much focus on treatment, not enough on preventing what makes us sick; too much focus on spurring economic development, not enough on taking care of what we've got."

    — ARMINE YALNIZYAN, economist and media commentator

"A very personal and passionate account from a doctor on the front lines of health care, this book should be required reading for every decision-maker in Canada."

    — GREG MARCHILDON, Ontario Research Chair in Health Policy
      and System Design

"*A Healthy Society* is an eloquent cry from the heart and a rational appeal to the mind. With meticulous research, dramatic personal histories, and precise analysis, Dr. Meili shows why our wealthy society is far from a healthy one. He illustrates how social status affects physical well-being and suggests steps necessary to create a culture that's democratic not only in the electoral sense but also in providing for the health of its members."

    — GABOR MATÉ, author of *In the Realm of Hungry Ghosts: Close Encounters*
      with Addiction

"Combining powerful analysis and compelling stories, Dr. Meili inspires us to engage in new politics to build a healthier, more equal society. May he continue to bring us together around bold ideas for change."

    — NIKI ASHTON, member of Parliament for Churchill–Keewatinook Aski

A HEALTHY SOCIETY

The author will donate
a portion of the proceeds from this book's sales
to Upstream and SWITCH.

Upstream is a movement to create a
healthy society through evidence-based, people centred ideas.
It seeks to reframe the public discourse around addressing
the social determinants of health.

SWITCH, the Student Wellness Initiative
Toward Community Health clinic, augments the training
of future professionals while improving the health, education,
and skills of people from Saskatoon's core communities.

Ryan Meili

A Healthy Society

How a Focus on Health Can Revive Canadian Democracy

UPDATED AND EXPANDED EDITION

PURICH
BOOKS

Purich Books, an imprint of UBC Press
2029 West Mall
Vancouver, BC, V6T 1Z2
www.purichbooks.ca

26 25 24 23 22 21 20 19   5 4

Printed in Canada on FSC ® certified ancient-forest-free paper
(100% post-consumer recycled) that is processed chlorine- and acid-free.

Library and Archives Canada Cataloguing in Publication

Meili, Ryan, author
A healthy society : how a focus on health can revive Canadian democracy /
Ryan Meili. – Updated and expanded edition.

Includes bibliographical references and index.
Issued in print and electronic formats.
ISBN 978-0-7748-8026-8 (softcover). – ISBN 978-0-7748-8027-5 (PDF). –
ISBN 978-0-7748-8028-2 (EPUB). – ISBN 978-0-7748-8029-9 (Kindle)

1. Health – Social aspects – Canada. 2. Health – Political aspects – Canada.
3. Public health – Political aspects – Canada. I. Title.

RA418.3.C3M44 2018   362.10971   C2017-906825-3
                                                       C2017-906826-1

Canadä

UBC Press gratefully acknowledges the financial support for our publishing
program of the Government of Canada (through the Canada Book Fund), the
Canada Council for the Arts, and the British Columbia Arts Council.

CONTENTS

FOREWORD

André Picard

In 1973, a fifteen-second public service announcement was broadcast showing a sixty-year-old Swede jogging effortlessly alongside a huffing and puffing thirty-year-old Canadian.

That PSA from ParticipACTION, although broadcast only six times, created an iconic image and sparked a national conversation on fitness, as well as massive investments in sport and recreation infrastructure.

The next year, 1974, then Minister of Health and Welfare Marc Lalonde issued his landmark report, *A New Perspective on the Health of Canadians*. It suggested that health should be considered distinct from medicine and that the "health field" should be broken into four broad areas: human biology, environment, lifestyle, and health care organization – in other words, "determinants of health exist outside of the health care systems."

While that message was more profound and potentially influential, it was greeted with a lot less enthusiasm than the "get fit" meme – at least in Canadian political circles and outside the confines of academia.

But other countries – particularly the Nordic countries, including Sweden – did take the Lalonde report philosophy to heart, recognizing that the best way to improve the health of their populations was to invest in social programs, not just sickness care.

Today, if we were to produce a PSA, the sixty-year-old Swede would still be more fit than his younger Canadian counterpart, but he would also live in a country where there is far less child poverty and homelessness, a better and more affordable education system, more progressive labour laws, more generous social welfare programs, decent social housing and progressive tax policies that ensure a much smaller gap between rich and poor, and a cheaper, more efficient sickness care system to boot.

Sweden is a striking example of the fact that the countries with the healthiest populations are those that have the least inequality.

A Healthy Society is, in many ways, the long-form version of that PSA. It explains, in plain language and with salient anecdotes, the importance of what academics call the social determinants of health.

When the book was first published five years ago, it was a breath of fresh air, a *cri de coeur* from a young social activist and aspiring politician.

Ryan Meili has come a long way since then. With the help of others, he founded Upstream, a national movement, and was elected as a Member of the Legislative Assembly of Saskatchewan, all the while continuing to practise medicine in Saskatoon's inner city and being active in a number of social causes, notably efforts to ensure refugees had access to health care.

In recent years, the debate about social determinants of health has also advanced in leaps and bounds, moving beyond academia to political circles, the media, and everyday discourse.

Thinking upstream – focusing on prevention and health promotion in the broadest sense of the terms – has, in many ways, gone mainstream.

That's probably because the concept is largely intuitive.

Stated plainly, it is not enough to patch people up when they are hurting and sick. We need to create the conditions that allow everyone to get and remain healthy in the first place.

That means ensuring everyone has a decent income, a roof over their heads, a good education, access to healthy food, a sound physical environment, a social environment free of racism and sexism, and a sense of belonging in their community.

It also means making a distinction between equality (treating everyone the same regardless of their needs) and equity (ensuring that everyone has what they need to be successful).

A just society embraces the latter.

In Canada, Indigenous peoples are the most glaring and visible victims of injustice and discrimination. After centuries of apartheid-like policies, we are beginning to recognize this truth and taking small steps toward reconciliation.

Efforts to improve the health of Indigenous peoples – or, more precisely, efforts to give First Nations, Inuit, and Métis peoples the ability to heal and rediscover their culture, languages, and healthy communities – have to be at the heart of that process.

No amount of medicine will allow those wounds to heal. But access to education, employment, housing, social programs, and a sound environment will accelerate a return to self-determination and salve some of the wounds of generations-long trauma.

The most powerful message of *A Healthy Society* is that the solution to economically costly societal ills like poverty is, above all, political.

Meili wears his politics on his sleeve – and that's refreshing. But it would be wrong to dismiss the ideas in this book as idealistic or, worse yet, left-wing.

Social determinants of health are not a leftist concept, nor are they the purview of socialists or liberals. Whether you believe in a "hand-up" or "handout" philosophy, the notion that our social and economic environment profoundly impacts our health is intuitive. And, whether you have left, right, or centrist political leanings, the concept that keeping people healthy is a better investment than trying to heal them later is inarguable.

So, there is much room for consensus, even in a broken political system, afflicted by too much partisanship and self-interest.

The challenge, of course, is turning the new-found understanding of social determinants of health into concrete policies and actions.

The uplifting message to be drawn from *A Healthy Society* is that creating a healthy society does not necessarily require grand gestures but, rather, a relentless focus on the basics.

FOREWORD
TO THE FIRST EDITION

Hon. Roy Romanow,
Former Premier of Saskatchewan

You hear it all the time – in the media, from the public, from politicians themselves: politics is broken. Canadians, and people around the world, are becoming increasingly frustrated with what they see as a widening chasm – a chasm between citizen values and public policy, between what people believe in and what governments do, between the world we envision and the one in which we live. There is a widespread belief, reflected in decreasing voter participation and growing cynicism among citizens, that the system isn't working as it should, that politicians aren't doing what they should. The question before us, as we hope for something better, is what exactly should they be doing?

For many years the primary measuring stick of societal success, and thus the primary goal of politicians, has been growth in Gross Domestic Product (GDP). By measuring economic activity, a growing GDP is thought to represent a thriving society. However, this measure is, by definition, insensitive to whether or not that economic activity contributes to the well-being of society. It counts things that harm us as well as those that improve our lives. The evidence against the use of GDP as a measurement is strong; it is clearly not a sufficient guide for our political actions. The problem facing policy makers, and disappointing the general population, is the lack of an accepted alternative.

Over the past decade or two, we've started to see the first signs of a significant transformation. There is, today, a growing international movement dedicated to redefining individual and societal well-being in a way that goes beyond simple measures of economic consumption. The fact is that trying to gauge societal progress by using GDP alone is like trying to use a slide rule to measure blood pressure – it may give you a number but it doesn't tell you a whole lot about well-being.

Financial stability is an important element of societal success, a necessary tool for achieving our goals. It is not, however, the true goal of a society. As Dr. Meili argues in the following pages, a far more meaningful goal is that of health. Health – that of our neighbours and friends, our families and ourselves – is something we all seek. It's also a far better measure of success than material wealth.

For this wiser goal to take precedence, however, we need a change in government attitudes. Governments of all stripes have to view the decisions they make through the prism of "will it invest in the well-being of our society – in our health and overall quality of life – or will it diminish those things?"

A promising means of assisting that change in attitude is a new method of measuring societal success, the Canadian Index of Wellbeing. This project, led by a pan-Canadian group of research experts and practitioners, has begun tracking and providing unique insights into the quality of life of Canadians in eight interconnected categories that truly matter: our standard of living; our health; the vitality of our communities; our education; the way we use our time; our participation in the democratic process; the state of our arts, culture, and recreation; and the quality of our environment. In October 2011, the first complete, numerical report of the Canadian Index of Wellbeing revealed that while Canada's GDP increased by 31 percent in the period between 1994 and 2008, the quality of life of Canadians improved by a mere 11 percent.

Aside from raising profound questions about the degree to which our economic prosperity is translating into better lives for Canadians, this report reaffirms earlier studies that demonstrate how closely linked well-being is to income and education levels. People with higher incomes and levels of education tend to live longer, are less likely to have diabetes and other chronic conditions, and are more likely to report excellent or very good health.

The stark reality is that household income continues to be one of the best predictors of future health status. The formula is straightforward:

more income equals better health, less income equals worse health. This is true in all age groups and for both women and men.

When we consider the impact of this reality on those at the lower end of the income scale, we realize that there exists a vicious cycle: poor people have more health problems. They need more medical services, but they can't afford them so they cut back on medications or diagnostic tests, or they pay for them by cutting back on other things like nutritious foods. This leads to more illness and lost time at work, which leads to lost income and jobs, which creates more poverty. The end result costs us all – financially through increased social costs and health care costs, but also in our ability to enjoy life in safe, vibrant communities.

It becomes increasingly clear that if we are ever to break this cycle, if we are ever to significantly reduce the enormous health inequities that exist in our society, then we must address the full range of key determinants that cause those inequities – economic determinants, social determinants, educational determinants, health care determinants, and environmental determinants, to name just a few.

Historians tell us that we have had two great revolutions in the course of public health. The first was the control of infectious diseases, notwithstanding some recent challenges. The second was the battle against non-communicable diseases. I believe that the third revolution is about moving from an illness model to focusing on all the things that both prevent illness and promote well-being. This third revolution, in which governments and citizens work together to address the determinants of health, will ensure that Canadians are the healthiest we can be. It will also set the stage for Canada once again to be a world leader in innovation for better health.

The impact of the social determinants of health is well known to governments and to health care organizations. The major challenge before us lies in turning this understanding into concrete actions that have an impact on individual Canadians and communities.

Too often our understanding of the ways in which income, education, and other living conditions determine health status is not translated into the policies and services that will lead to change. We have not made the transition into a political system that creates the circumstances in which people can thrive, in which they can enjoy the fullness of well-being.

Rather, there are many millions of people who continue to suffer from illness and die far too young due to the disconnect between our knowledge and our action.

The ideas confirmed by those who have studied the determinants of health, including the researchers who have developed the Canadian Index of Wellbeing, need desperately to be translated into the public pressure and political will required to bring about the third revolution in public health.

A revolution cannot happen without those individuals who are willing to take the risks to provoke lasting change, to turn ideas into action. If this third revolution is to take place, these leaders must articulate the vision of a healthy society in a way that people will find at once meaningful and motivating. Dr. Meili's experiences as a clinician give him an up-close view of the determinants of health in the lives of his patients. His passion for their plight brings a sense of immediacy to his cries for change. His personal experience, both political and medical, gives him the outlook needed to propose practical solutions.

More than a voice for those who go too often unheard, *A Healthy Society* proposes a new approach to organizing for change. The stories of those most affected by the determinants of health breathe life into a reasoned argument for a system more responsive to their needs. The proposed focus for that system, the health of us all, offers us a common goal that everyone, regardless of their position in society, can support. *A Healthy Society* offers an inspiring means to fix what is broken in Canadian politics.

Saskatoon, 2012

PREFACE

The protection of the people's health should be
recognized by the government as its primary obligation
and duty to its citizens.

– Norman Bethune[1]

A man as thin as a skeleton sits coughing in a tent near the hospital la-
trine, patiently taking his tuberculosis treatment and hoping he doesn't
have a drug-resistant strain. A father's support makes all the difference
for a young woman struggling to stay off street drugs while waiting for
cancer treatment. A five-month-old girl the size of a newborn is brought
into hospital by her father, who has been feeding her canned milk since
her mother died. An elderly man is sent to a nursing home an hour's
drive away from where he's lived with his wife for sixty years; they can't
manage at home with his dementia, and there are no long-term spaces
available nearby. Having lost their home to flooding, a family wonders
how it will care for a physically disabled child. A Dene elder goes into
a diabetic coma and dies at home, waiting for the ambulance that was
busy with a car accident on the gravel road leading to her reserve. A
doctor in a wealthy suburb prescribes an anti-depressant to a man who
has been having trouble sleeping and concentrating; she wonders
whether she should be taking them as well. Having lost his job due to

an economic downturn, a middle-aged man is forced to choose between his children's school fees and his blood pressure medication.

Income, education, employment, housing, the wider environment, and social supports: these, far more than the actions of physicians, nurses, and other health care providers, have the most impact on our health. If Norman Bethune was correct, and the greatest role of government is protecting the health of the population, it is in these areas that our public policy must have its strongest emphasis.

In *A Healthy Society*, the stories of patient experiences lead into a discussion of health and its role in determining our political direction, our collective decisions. With health as a commonly held goal, the drive for better human health can be a shared mission for society. When people understand what really makes a difference in our health – the determinants of health – they realize how great a role politics play in deciding the health of everyone. A renewed focus on health offers hope to change a political climate that has bred skepticism and mistrust among Canadians.

I begin with the case for putting health front and centre in our public discourse – in how we organize politically, in how we plan, and in how we judge the success of our actions and our political representatives. Before doing so, I pause briefly in the field of medicine and the health sciences to explore some emerging ideas that could be usefully applied to politics and to discuss the growing advocacy movement among health care providers. We then examine the current predominant focus for our society, that of economic well-being, and take a deeper look at its converse of poverty. This is followed by the exploration of the specific health determinants, connecting patient stories with the policies that could create the conditions for better health. The final section discusses the democratic reforms that could help reshape the way we organize ourselves to create a truly healthy society.

The original version of *A Healthy Society*, published in 2012 by Purich Publishing in Saskatoon, sold over five thousand copies across Canada. It also informed the development of Upstream, a national non-profit organization promoting understanding of and action on the social determinants of health. It took me across the country, speaking to audiences of health care providers, political leaders, and the general public on the ideas within and learning from the people directly involved in the health equity movement. It also saw me move from practising medicine and teaching at the University of Saskatchewan to trying to apply these ideas as an elected Member of the Legislative Assembly in Saskatchewan.

In the five years since the first edition, the public understanding of the social determinants of health has grown, and I've learned a great deal more about communicating these ideas. This new edition includes updated information in each of the original chapters. There is a new chapter on advocacy and another on a new approach to addressing poverty. The original chapter on housing, food security, and the environment has been separated into two to give a more detailed treatment of these issues.

Sir Michael Marmot has called for a "social movement, based on evidence, to reduce inequalities in health."[2] It is my hope that this book can contribute to sharing the evidence and advancing the social movement for healthy politics in Canada.

A HEALTHY SOCIETY

1

A HEALTHY SOCIETY

> The development of a society, rich or poor, can
> be judged by the quality of its population's health,
> how fairly health is distributed across the social
> spectrum, and the degree of protection provided
> from disadvantage as a result of ill-health.
>
> – Commission on Social Determinants of Health,
> *Closing the Gap in a Generation*[1]

Buying Smokes for My Patients

Maxine just turned twenty, but she walks like she's ninety-one. I suppose that's because she's closer to death than most ninety-one-year-olds. You'd walk slowly, too, if that's what lay ahead. She's been on the street since she was thirteen, hooked on IV cocaine and morphine for nearly as long, but she's had HIV for only two years, three at the most. For some reason, like many of the growing number of people in Saskatchewan who are infected with HIV, she is a "rapid progresser." This means that her infection didn't take years to progress to the immune suppression of AIDS. It happened very quickly. There are a few theories as to why this occurs: different genetic capacity to respond, unique strains of the virus, or simply poor underlying health. The truth is, we don't quite know why. What we do know is that she's in really bad shape – what

3

many doctors would call, in back rooms and unprofessional asides, a train wreck.

When I first met Maxine, she came in with florid thrush, a rip-roaring pneumonia, and a prescription for prophylactic antibiotics that she never intended to fill. I instantly recalled the hospital in Mozambique, where caring for young men and women who arrived emaciated and scared, fast approaching the end of their lives, was a daily occurrence. Maxine's is the worst case of AIDS I've seen walking a Canadian street. I told her she was sick enough to go into hospital, but she had just been discharged for the umpteenth time. She wouldn't say much, just told me she wanted antibiotics and nutritional supplements. The last thing she wanted was to go back into the hospital.

Three months later, the word on the street is that Maxine wants help. She's getting weaker and sicker, and finally recognizes she's in trouble. She comes into the clinic and falls asleep on the exam table. She is deathly thin, and under my stethoscope her lungs sound like a rubber boot being pulled from the mud. I call the infectious disease service and internal medicine at Royal University Hospital. They know her well; she's done this before. She gets sick enough to need help, is admitted, gets a bit better, hates the hospital, misses the drugs, and bolts. Reluctantly, they agree to give her another try.

That was a Friday, and I was out of town for the weekend. When I arrived to see her on Monday morning, the internal medicine team was about to discharge her. Her CD4 count, a measure of the immune cells that defend against infection, is 4. It should be at least 400. The HIV viral load tells us how active the virus is in her system. More than 100,000 is considered too much; hers is 3 million. However, her pneumonia has improved, she's not ready for the anti-retroviral medications that must be taken every day to avoid increasing resistance, and she is no longer sick enough that she needs to be on the acute ward. She doesn't make it easy to help her, either. She swears at the nurses, refuses to take pills or have blood work. When the security guard assigned to keep her in line takes her for walks, she bums cigarettes, hides them in her gown, and smokes them on the ward. She takes as much time and attention as the rest of the patients on her ward combined, and the nurses and medical staff are exasperated.

Despite her misbehaviour, she tells me she wants to stay. I visit twice a day, sitting on the edge of her bed and talking with her about the future. She says she wants to get on methadone and off the streets. She wants to take the anti-retroviral medications to start her immune system working again. She is refusing to leave the hospital. The idea that, as health care providers, we might have security guards escort this young girl who is dying of AIDS to the street is against all we stand for.

So we don't. After a long discussion with the medical team, we agree to try a little longer. Give her a week and see how she does. Because, despite the frustrations of bed shortages, extra workload, and chances that are cachectically slim, we know these are the moments that define us as a profession. Even when the odds are long, we cannot walk away from someone who is so clearly suffering. So we'll try for another week. Get the methadone doc to see her, get psychiatry involved, and social work, and nutrition, and anyone else we can think of; make our boundaries clear and try once more.

We know the hospital is no place for Maxine. But the system has no better place. Most drug rehab programs won't take people on methadone; none of them will take someone who needs to start it. The waiting list to get into a program can be several months and requires people with numerous social and economic barriers to jump through multiple hoops that seem designed to keep them out. So in the gap between wanting to kick the drugs and having the personal and social capacity to do so, they're dumped back on the streets to start from scratch.

On the second or third night of this experiment in patience, I go up to see Maxine. The nurses are frustrated; she's still sneaking smokes into her room. She constantly demands that security take her for walks. She fights meds and blood work. But she's still there. She's taking her methadone. She tells me again she wants to stay; she wants to get better. The nurses think that maybe if she had her own cigarettes, they could help her set a schedule for when to have one and help her stay out of the trouble she finds when she leaves the hospital. Maybe if they print off more of the crossword puzzles she likes, she'll keep busy. In many ways she is older than her twenty years. In others, she's truly a child.

The next morning I go in to see her. I've got a couple of books of crossword puzzles and a pack of Player's Light. I never thought I'd buy a pack of smokes for a patient, but in this case "first do no harm" takes a back seat to the immediate fight for her life. I go up to her room to deliver my gifts and talk with her. She's gone. The night before, she got frustrated, left the hospital, scored some drugs, shot up, and showed up in emergency in bad shape. The line was crossed and she is no longer welcome in the hospital. She can come to see me at the clinic the next week – we'll always see her – but the glimmer of hope is significantly dulled.

The last time I saw her, just before I stopped working at the clinic she trusts, she was repeatedly wearing out her welcome at the brief detox centre near the clinic. I told her I hoped she'd at least come in and take her medications and see the other doctors there. She said goodbye, and thank you, and gave me a heartbreakingly innocent hug.

The cigarettes stayed in my freezer for a long time. I thought maybe the next time I was invited to a sweat lodge ceremony, I'd bring them as my offering of tobacco and say a prayer for Maxine. It turned out I didn't get the chance – at least not while she was still alive. A few weeks after I left the clinic to work in rural Saskatchewan, a car hit her, shattering her pelvis. While in hospital she contracted pneumonia again, and this time she couldn't recover from it. She died just before her twenty-second birthday.

It's easy to get fixated on the pathology of Maxine's story, to think that it's about viral invasion, fractured bones, and infected lungs. These physical details, however, are distractions from the real disease. They are symptoms of what Stu Skinner, a Saskatoon infectious disease physician who specializes in HIV, refers to as the "End Stage of Poverty." Maxine's life was hard from the beginning. She grew up in an environment of poverty, dysfunction, and abuse. Her mother had spent most of her own childhood in a residential school; she hadn't seen what it was like to be a parent and wasn't very good at it. Maxine never knew her father. Instead, she knew the attentions of various boyfriends and extended family members who abused her physically, sexually, and emotionally throughout her childhood. She had a baby before she reached Grade 9 and never returned to finish high school. In many ways she never got a chance to be a child, and at the same time never matured to be an adult.

Such a broken life, such an inherently tragic existence, provokes serious questions about our society: questions about the prevention and treatment of disease, about poverty and services for vulnerable people, about education, and about justice. What often escapes our attention when we consider the tragic story of one individual is how intimately it is connected to all of us, to the collective decision-making process that is electoral politics. It is politics that decide whether young women like Maxine live or die. Ultimately, our political choices are to blame for the large number of people who slip through the cracks.

There is strong evidence that our current political choices aren't working for everyone. In Canada and around the world, the health of the poorest people is far worse than that of the richest, and new evidence suggests that we all suffer as a result. If we are to address the fundamental unfairness of this situation, we need to rethink not just how we do health care, but how we make decisions as a society.

Economic growth and advances in health care have improved human longevity, health status, and quality of life all over the world. Yet there are many people, in both poor countries and rich ones, who do not experience the benefits of this progress. Canada is one of the wealthiest nations on the planet, but the gap between the rich and the poor is widening, and rates of child poverty and homelessness are rising. Despite Canada's self-image as a welcoming and equal place, Indigenous people, immigrants, and women continue to suffer more illness than the rest of the population. The cost of post-secondary education has become unaffordable for many. Epidemics of drug abuse, diabetes, obesity, HIV/AIDS, and other diseases closely related to poverty result in lost lives and wounded communities. Meanwhile, human actions are harming the wider environment that supports life; this, in turn, harms humans. These problems are fundamentally political, but those who object to the current state of affairs, who suggest that there must be a better way of organizing ourselves for the benefit of all, are dismissed as naïve and ignorant of economic realities.

None of this is news. Most people are well aware of the situation, and many are moved to action. Their overall response, however, is fragmented, confused, and ineffective. The question before us is how can we move beyond this impasse? How can we organize ourselves to make wise decisions that will benefit everyone?

Politics and public discourse, the field that should be responding to such pressing societal concerns, flounders instead from crisis to crisis. Parties and public figures bounce around the political and social spectrum in reaction to events or public opinion. The key issues of the day are decided more by the news cycle than by any rational understanding of priorities. Ideas are presented by extreme opposite views in debate rather than in a search for common ground. Political reporting is dominated by scandal to the exclusion of substance, and as a result, we are unable to focus on real issues. The agenda of governments seems to be either hidden or absent. From day to day, the top stories change from an international conflict to a far-off natural disaster, from the rising or falling loonie to a record lottery jackpot, with no discernible pattern of progress or failure. In this fragmented experience of history and the present, we all have a hard time recognizing what is really happening, what a government has done, or what it ought to do.

The problem is not a failure to understand the extent of our difficulties; it is the lack of a focus, of an organizing principle for change. An undeclared objective will not be realized; we must state our goals clearly if we wish to reach them. In the absence of a societal project that advances the well-being of all, it is only natural that groups will use politics cynically for their own gains and that people will find it difficult to decipher the mixed and ever-changing signals. Without clear common goals, we have increasing polarity and discord. If we are to make anything of this mess, we must find something we agree on and work toward it. We need a clear objective that will inspire people from diverse circumstances to work together for a greater good.

Windows and Frames

The roots of our most significant health problems are not clinical: they are social, political. This means that the solutions must be political as well. Public opinion determines, as it should in a democracy, what solutions are available. But what determines public opinion?

At any given moment, there is a range of acceptable and desirable ideas, with others lying outside the realm of possibility. This is sometimes referred to as Overton's Window – the policy options that politicians can safely discuss without being considered too radical to be elected.[2] The window changes over time, with marriage between same-sex couples being a recent example of something that was unthinkable only a few decades ago but is now widely accepted.[3]

Like all windows, that of political possibility is delimited and determined by its frame. As George Lakoff, author of *Don't Think of an Elephant!*, famously notes, "all politics is moral."[4] Much more than a cold, rational analysis of arguments and statistics, frames are the moral lenses we use to decide what policies and politicians to support. They refer to our deep understanding of issues and, though not solely about language, can be greatly influenced by the way in which an issue is described or discussed. Language choice determines which moral frame is activated and – depending on people's underlying values – which policy they are likely to support.

The terms of debate, and the window of possibilities, are defined by the active frame. Imagine you have a friend who is paranoid of the coming zombie apocalypse. He tells you of the many steps he's taken to protect his house from attacks. You don't believe in zombies, but in arguing with him, you highlight the weaknesses of his defences, explaining that the undead will merely come in through his garage or that he'll never get to the shotguns under the bed in time. By accepting his framing, you've lost the argument from the beginning.

Now, that's a bit of a silly example, but we are constantly dealing with frames that, despite being countered repeatedly with arguments and evidence, continue to rise from the grave. We see economic growth presented as the most important political objective, rather than a necessary means to the greater end of improving our lives. We see framing that all taxes are a burden and any tax cut a relief, rather than talking about taxation as an essential tool for funding social investment. Frames of austerity in a time of abundance, of the private sector as the sole source of efficiency and innovation, of the poor being to blame for their own circumstances, all of these limit our ability to think differently about the problems before us and to seek the most creative means of addressing them.

The way to move the window is not to argue with the existing frames, it's to put forward a new one, to allow ourselves to focus on what really matters. What I propose is that we already have that new frame, that people have already chosen the focus. It is simply a matter of recognizing, understanding, articulating, and acting upon it. The focus is health: the health of individuals, the health of communities, the health of democratic institutions.

People care about health. It's part of our assumed common ground, a truly shared value that transcends class, colour, and political ideology. We greet people by asking how they are, asking about their well-being. The conversations that follow are replete with references to health. We speak of healthy relationships, healthy attitudes, healthy economies, and healthy appetites. We toast each other's health. If you ask expectant parents whether they're having a boy or a girl, the answer is inevitably, "We don't care, as long as they're healthy." When neighbours and friends are ill, we go out of our way to help them. If people fall on hard times, a common encouragement is, "At least you have your health." These familiar expressions reflect our unconscious preoccupation with our common vulnerabilities, hopes, and fears: we know, deeply, that good health – physical, mental, and social – is a necessary condition for the full enjoyment of life.

This focus on health is reflected in public life as well, particularly in the heated political debates around health care and health spending. Health care and health are very different things, but health care is the policy area most obviously linked to health, and the attention given to it is an identifiable surrogate for this deeper preoccupation. With rare exceptions, health care is the number-one issue of importance in Canadian polling, an unusual constant in the tumultuous sea of public opinion. Polls taken during federal elections since the mid-1990s have consistently ranked health care as the issue of greatest importance to voters, more so than employment, debt, taxation, and the environment.[5] Accordingly, health care takes up the largest portion of provincial budgets. Many people have complained about this, asserting that an inordinate focus on health takes away from other important areas such as education, justice, and infrastructure. In a way they're right – our focus on health care at the expense of other key aspects of public life is disproportionate. But the problem is not that we care too much about health: it's that we are doing so in an incomplete and reactive fashion.

The reality is that health is already 100 percent of the budget. If we understood that, we would make better choices. Decisions in and across all ministries – education, environment, finance, justice, and so on – all influence health outcomes. There are opportunities in every sector of government to improve health and prevent illness. Our approach tends to be palliative rather than preventative; we focus too much on what to do when our health fails, not on how to ensure that we thrive and stay healthy. If we truly want a healthy society, we need to build a political movement with health as its focus.

So Urban It's Rural

To explore the idea of health as a focus for public discourse, I'll start with an example, one that hits very close to home for me. I live in Saskatoon, a city of nearly a quarter million people on the Canadian prairie. My house is in a neighbourhood called Riversdale, a few blocks west of the South Saskatchewan River. Riversdale is one of five core neighbourhoods that make up this part of town, often referred to simply as the west side. Some people are surprised that a small urban centre such as Saskatoon should have an inner city, but it certainly does, with all its accompanying charms and difficulties. My neighbours keep an eye on the house when I'm away, and in summer they share fresh carrots and zucchini from their gardens. Strangers lean over the hedge to chat when I'm out raking leaves. People greet me with "Hi, Doc" when we pass on the street. I often say it's so urban it's rural.

Though the isolation of the core neighbourhoods amid the city's doughnut development (with peripheral suburbs and big box stores pulling social and economic activity away from the centre) has conferred upon them some small-town charms, their problems are decidedly urban. These neighbourhoods have the lowest per capita income in Saskatoon. They have a reputation for petty and violent crime, and are an active marketplace for illicit drugs and prostitution. They are also plagued by a significant deficit in services, including frequent shortages of quality housing, access to good nutrition (there has been no real grocery store in the area for years), health services, and more. As a result, the health of their residents is the worst in the city.

The fate of Station 20 West is typical of the way in which these communities have been treated. In the spring of 2007, the Saskatchewan government dedicated $8 million to this innovative project, a collaboration between community groups in the core neighbourhoods, with the goal of addressing service gaps and creating economic opportunities. Community-based organizations such as CHEP Good Food and Quint, a housing co-op based in the five neighbourhoods, joined with the Saskatoon Community Clinic, the University of Saskatchewan, and the Saskatoon Health Region to design this unique response. The name, Station 20 West, played off its location, literally just on the wrong side of the tracks crossing 20th Street, the core's main drag. Billed as the "Engine of Urban Renewal," it featured a wide variety of services and community development initiatives in one convenient location.

Station 20 West was to be situated next to fifty-six new affordable housing units and a branch of the public library. It was to include a dental outreach clinic, a community health clinic, a student-run after-hours clinic, offices for the aforementioned community-based organizations and others (including Heifer International and the Elizabeth Fry Society), a university outreach education centre, and a member-owned co-op grocery store called the Good Food Junction. These were all to be housed in a building that would set a standard for environmentally responsible development, with the highest level of LEED (Leadership in Energy and Environmental Design) certification.

At least, that was the plan. In the November 2007 provincial election, the governing New Democratic Party (NDP) was defeated by the Saskatchewan Party. In March 2008, the new government informed Station 20 West board members that the dedicated funds were being rescinded. Just months before starting construction, the project's future seemed extremely dim. The new government's ill-considered decision to withdraw its funding shocked the people of Saskatoon, triggering a firestorm of criticism and a groundswell of support for the project. In April 2008, in one of the largest demonstrations that Saskatchewan had seen in decades, over 2,500 people from across the city took to the streets to proclaim their support for Station 20 West. Despite this show of support, funding was not reinstated, and the organizers had to start from scratch.

At the time, I was a family physician in the clinic that was slated to relocate to Station 20 West. While working on the west side as a student, a resident in family medicine, and later as a practising family doctor, I had become quite excited about the potential of this project and was deeply disappointed when its funding was cancelled.

Clinical work in underserved areas offers many joys: the sense of community, the easy humour and relaxed attitude of many patients, and for me a sense of purpose, as I am often able to connect with people in real need and offer them meaningful support. When I was first planning to study medicine, I had a naïve notion that what doctors did was make friends all day. Patients come in, you hear their stories, help as best you can, and make a connection. After a decade of practise, with time in northern Saskatchewan and all over the rural areas of the province, rural Mozambique, and inner-city Saskatoon, that's exactly how it feels. The questions we're asked aren't easy, and people aren't always pleased with the answers, but all-in-all that's exactly what the job is: making friends all day.

As such, it's extremely rewarding, but it's also very frustrating. I want the best for my patients, my friends, but every day I see patients whose problems are not merely physical. They're political. They stem from a lack of safe or appropriate housing, a lack of education, or simply from not having enough money to afford the basic necessities of life. People don't get sick when they come into the clinic or show up at the hospital; their problems can't be solved there, either. They get sick in their real lives: at home, at school, at work, and at play.

Healthy, Wealthy, and Why

The notion that health and illness are determined by life circumstances is not new, and in recent years it has become a staple of health theory and teaching. In one of the first lectures of medical school, students are asked to name the greatest factors that decide whether someone will be healthy or ill. They commonly mention lifestyle choices, such as the so-called holy trinity of diet, exercise, and smoking cessation.[6] Some talk about access to health services, and others cite genetics or culture. After this discussion, the students are shown a list of health determinants such as this one from the Canadian Institute for Health Information. In order of impact, the twelve factors that make the biggest difference in people's health are

- income status
- education
- social support networks
- employment and working conditions
- early childhood development
- physical environment
- personal health practices and coping skills
- biological and genetic factors
- health services
- gender
- culture
- mass media technology (i.e., TV viewing and physical inactivity).[7]

Invariably, this list comes as something of a surprise to students. As aspiring doctors, they think they are getting into the business of making people healthy. Then they see that the services offered by the health professions barely crack the top ten.

The lesson to be drawn from the list of determinants, and the one that is stressed to students, is that the most important factors that determine health are social, and the most effective solutions are political. Health services have much less effect on ultimate health outcomes than social determinants such as income and education, housing and nutrition. Gender, culture, and biology, the more immutable of the determinants, also figure near the bottom. What the students learn is that, though they may indeed have the power to heal, they cannot act alone. The response to illness is not limited to one profession or sector: it must be societal.

The question, then, is where does it make the most sense to focus our political efforts? In other words, which determinants of health are most directly affected by public policy? There are many lists of social determinants of health in Canada, but the most commonly used cites them as income and income distribution, education, unemployment and job security, employment and working conditions, early childhood development, food insecurity, housing, social exclusion, social safety net, health services, Aboriginal status, gender, race, and disability.[8] As you can see, these are all areas where public policy can change a person's situation or experience to either improve or worsen health. If optimal health is the desired destination, this list is the road map of where to invest to reach that goal.

When we address inadequate housing, when we stop gender discrimination and racism, when we ensure that people have work that is safe and fair, and that our children receive the care and attention they need to grow, we can dramatically improve health outcomes. So what's holding us back?

An Unhealthy Imbalance

The list of social determinants rings true to me and to others who work with the people of Saskatoon's west side. Most of our patients are First Nations or Métis. We also see many refugees and other newcomers. They face challenges in accessing child care and education. Unemployment, poverty, and dependence on an inadequate social safety net are endemic, particularly for women. Housing is expensive and often crowded or unsafe. Health care services are limited and difficult to access. Violence, racism, sexual exploitation, and substance abuse are only a few of the many symptoms of ongoing poverty and social exclusion. The list goes on, and the result is ill health.

The effects of the social determinants on health are readily apparent to those who live and work in underserved communities. They are also supported by studies such as "Health Disparity by Neighbourhood Income," a 2006 article in the *Canadian Journal of Public Health*.[9] This study compared the health of the six lowest-income neighbourhoods in Saskatoon (according to Statistics Canada) with the same health indicators in the rest of the city. The findings were startling. People in the core were four times more likely to have diabetes, four to seven times more likely to get a sexually transmitted illness, and fifteen times more likely to have hepatitis C. Those in the core also experienced significantly higher rates of injury, mental illness, and coronary artery disease.

When the six poorest neighbourhoods were compared with the city's six most affluent areas, the contrast was greater still. People who lived in the core were fifteen times more likely to contract a sexually transmitted infection, fifteen times more likely to attempt suicide, thirty-five times more likely to get hepatitis C, and thirteen times more likely to have type 2 diabetes than those who lived in the suburbs. Children in the core were half as likely to have received their vaccinations. With all these increased risks, a core neighbourhood resident was 2.5 times more likely to die in any given year. The infant mortality rate was three times higher in the lowest-income neighbourhoods than in the more affluent ones.

To get a sense of income ratios, the average family income in the six core neighbourhoods was approximately $30,000 per year, in the rest of Saskatoon it was over $60,000, and in the wealthiest areas it was just under $100,000.[10] Forty-four percent of families in the core live below the low-income cut-off line, compared with less than 4 percent among their high-income counterparts. People from the wealthier neighbourhoods are more than five times as likely to have progressed past Grade 9 or to have current employment. This landmark study revealed the huge disparities in health in Saskatoon and the obvious correlation to the social determinants.

Since that time, many other studies across Canada and around the world have demonstrated similar results. For example, if you live in the North End of Winnipeg, you're likely to die sixteen years earlier than other residents in the city.[11] In Hamilton, the Code Red project showed a difference in life expectancy of twenty-one years between the wealthiest and poorest neighbourhoods.[12]

A 2016 update of the Saskatoon study, led by Dr. Cory Neudorf, compared health outcomes to levels of income across Saskatchewan.[13] One of the most striking findings was how much inequality had increased in recent years. Between 2001 and 2011, income had gone up by seven dollars for the highest 20 percent of earners for every dollar it had risen for those in the lowest 20 percent. In that same period, housing and food prices jumped considerably, meaning that the basics of life were less afford-able. As the income gap widened, so did the outcome gap. The lowest-earning group saw a steady increase in mortality rates, with 50 percent more deaths in 2009 as compared to 2001.

Saskatchewan has a reputation for seeking equality, particularly with regard to health. It was the first province to institute what would even-tually become Medicare, a national health insurance program designed to ensure that all Canadians would receive care based on need rather than ability to pay. It is also a reasonably well-off province in one of the wealthiest and supposedly most advanced countries of the world. The discordance between perception and the reality of the drastic imbalance in health has been a shocking embarrassment for Saskatchewan. It is, paradoxically, not particularly surprising. We know, and have known for a long time, that poverty is the greatest contributor to ill health. What is new about these studies is the way in which they quantify our assump-tions, showing in simple and clear data that the effect is much larger than most people would have predicted or any could possibly justify. And the implications are obvious, though politically inconvenient: one, poverty and inequality kill; two, governments that stand idly by are complicit in every avoidable illness and premature death.

Waking Up Democracy

This embarrassment and shock could serve as a wake-up call. It could help to refocus our political discourse on the real work of a democracy. Our job, as people who govern ourselves, is to strive to do so in a way that is fair and good, that allows everyone to participate fully and enjoy wisely the good things given to us by providence. A functioning dem-ocracy is one in which the government, to the best of its ability, carries out the will of the people and takes seriously its responsibility to serve the best interests of all citizens. This democratic governance requires a number of things, key among them being that people are sufficiently informed to articulate their real needs, sufficiently empowered to present them as demands that can't be ignored, and sufficiently organized to see the process through to fruition. To put it another way, a democratic society requires a shared notion of what is good and a willingness to find a way to reach it. This does not imply that everyone would agree on all points and would work together in constant harmony. Democracy is the messy, argumentative, painstaking art of navigating a common course among conflicting priorities; if it isn't, we can be sure that some voices aren't being heard. Or, as one colleague in the world of HIV advocacy said to me, "If your coalition is comfortable, it's not broad enough." Having some shared framework, some set of guiding principles to steer the course, helps these differing priorities to be weighed by all in terms of what is best for all.

I mentioned earlier the importance we give, in private and in public, to human health. The World Health Organization defines health as "a state of complete physical, mental and social well-being and not merely the absence of disease or infirmity."[14] We all want health for ourselves and our family. The role of government in a democracy is to work with the people to produce what they want and need. What better goal for a society than to ensure that everyone enjoys true health – a state of complete physical, mental, and social well-being? And what better measure of the success of a government, and the society it represents, than the health of the people?

If we as a society address the social determinants of health – economy, education, the environment, and more – people will enjoy fuller, healthier lives. This much is clear: the road map of the social determinants can guide us to that shining shared goal of health for all. If we are transparent in our intentions, decisive in our actions, and honest in our evaluation of the results, we will also foster a common purpose that deepens community, builds solidarity, and rejuvenates democracy. In short, we will have found a means to move beyond our fragmented, haphazard approach to governance to one that works.

Yet some will object to such an approach. Change is hard, especially if it comes with a cost. If people doubt that they will benefit from it, they will be resistant. Any reasonable approach to building a healthy society, especially one informed by social accountability or social justice, means that improving conditions among the poorest residents must be a top priority. The foundation of a healthy society must be built among those who find themselves at the bottom. We need to move beyond a focus on equality to one that stresses equity, from treating people as if they are exactly the same regardless of their circumstances to responding to their real needs in order to achieve the best possible outcome It is by using an equity approach and directing our resources to the most marginalized that addressing the determinants of health will have the greatest impact: for those who are directly affected and, perhaps paradoxically or counter-intuitively, for everyone in society.

There are many people who see the world through compassionate eyes, who are motivated by a sense of social justice and who act altruistic-ally to improve the world. However, many of us don't follow suit; perhaps we don't enjoy the luxury of doing so. We look first to the needs of our family, to a little more enjoyment of our own existence. We are guided by rational self-interest, and we support the politicians who share our world view, who offer us a little more money in our pockets or protection from the forces that threaten our peace and security. What we fail to recognize is that it is in the best interests of everyone, even those at the top, to improve the health of all.

Helping Some Helps Us All

Addressing the social determinants of health doesn't just help those who are most in need; it helps everyone, regardless of social position. This is why the concept is so important: everyone benefits. This approach can be used to reach across divisions of class, race, geography, or political affiliation. The poverty and ill health of some affect us all. Poverty is a drag on the economy. When people live in poverty, they are unable to participate fully in public life and the marketplace, and cannot contrib-ute to the common account through taxes. They are also more likely to require health services, fall into the prison system, or need social assist-ance. People who lack decent housing or access to education are less able to participate in the economy as customers, workers, or innovators. As their health suffers, the costs are borne by taxpayers. Our jails are not filled with hardened criminals (at least, not when they go in); the vast majority of crimes against property and people stem from poverty. Our safety, prosperity, and satisfaction with society are decreased by gross inequality.

In *The Spirit Level: Why More Equal Societies Almost Always Do Better*, epidemiologists Richard Wilkinson and Kate Pickett present compelling evidence that the degree to which resources are unequally distributed has a significant impact on the health of everyone.[15] Countries with higher levels of equality, such as Japan or the Scandinavian nations, have much better health outcomes overall than countries with higher levels of inequality, such as the United States or Britain. Although the ill effects of inequality are greater for those at the bottom of the social ladder, the impact is not limited to the poorest few. Health outcomes follow a gradient of wealth: the working poor have worse health than the middle class, whose health is not as good as that of higher-earning professionals, and so on up the social and economic scale. But even the wealthiest people in an unequal society are less healthy than they would be in a more equal one. Whether it is the stress of constant competition and jockeying for position, the threat of personal ruin, or the burden of a large, marginalized population on public services and the social fabric, there is something about the experience of living in a society with a vast gap between rich and poor that damages everyone's health, resulting in more mental and physical illness, shorter lives, greater levels of obesity, and higher infant mortality. Less equal societies suffer more of the social problems that lead to negative health effects, experiencing higher levels of violence, imprisonment, illiteracy, and teen pregnancy.

Living in a more egalitarian country, on the other hand, benefits the health of everyone, from the least advantaged to the most successful. The editors of the *British Medical Journal* grasped the significance of these findings: "The big idea is that what matters in determining mortality and health in a society is less the overall wealth of that society and more how evenly that wealth is distributed. The more equally wealth is distributed, the better the health of that society."[16]

Any serious attempt to address health disparities must therefore involve a plan to address not just poverty, but wealth disparity as well.

This is not an easy idea to sell, especially not in countries that have a strong systemic commitment to inequality. But if, as the Commission on Social Determinants of Health's *Closing the Gap* report asserts, ill health is caused by the inequitable distribution of power, money, and resources,[17] any serious attempt to address health inequities must involve a plan to distribute resources more fairly.

The common response to stories of people living in poverty is that they are poor because of their own bad choices. Individuals who succeed in life possess the drive, determination, and skills to get ahead; they make wise decisions. If we look back at Maxine, there's no denying that she didn't make the wisest of decisions. The question is, could she have done differently?

To choose well, one needs to have had the chance – through good role models, through childhood development, through access to the basic necessities of life – to have developed some real wisdom. Maxine didn't choose the life she was born into, and that life didn't equip her to make better choices than she did. In fact – through poverty, abuse, lack of education, discrimination, and social exclusion – it worked against her at every step. It's hard to imagine anyone succeeding in her circumstances. Although we can't create a system that can force people to make wise choices, we can work toward one where more people have the opportunity to do so. By making the social determinants of health a primary driver of public policy, we can develop a society in which more people have the chance to succeed and to live better lives as a result. We can create the conditions that allow for good choices.

Providing everyone the opportunity to improve their lives, to escape poverty and experience the fullness of health, is not just the right thing to do, but also the smart thing to do. It is a delightful coincidence that our future well-being depends not on our selfishness but on our generosity, our sense of justice. The growing gap between rich and poor impoverishes us all, diminishing the quality of life for rich and poor alike. We in Canada consider ourselves a developed country, but to allow the gulf between rich and poor to expand is to become less developed.

The dream of a truly healthy society offers us a shared goal with the power to reach across the differences that separate us. It allows us to connect with our neighbours in recognition of our common vulnerability and our common desire to lead full and healthy lives. By systematically addressing the determinants of health and continually measuring our success, we can do both what is right and what is smart. We can chart a path of meaningful progress. We can improve the health of people and of the political system at the same time.

2
MEDICINE ON
A LARGER SCALE

Medicine is a social science, and politics is nothing more
than medicine on a large scale.

– Rudolf Virchow, *Collected Essays on Public Health
and Epidemiology*, 1848[1]

Rudolf Virchow was a pioneer in the field of pathology. Every medical
student learns about Virchow's node, a growth above the collarbone that
signifies stomach cancer. At some point in their studies, they are sure to
be quizzed on Virchow's triad, the three changes within veins that can
cause blood clots. What fewer students know is that, as well as being the
prolific scientist behind these eponyms, he was a prominent nineteenth-
century German politician and one of the first to write in depth on what
are now referred to as the social determinants of health. He was also an
early advocate of public health, stating that physicians, because of their
constant exposure to the unequal distribution of sickness and premature
death, should be the "natural attorneys of the poor."[2]

Among his writings was the introductory quote to this chapter, a
justification for dividing his time between his practice as a pathologist
and his political work. The idea that politics are medicine on a larger
scale is one that influenced me not only to become directly involved in
the political process, but also to seek what political lessons might be
gleaned from the diverse study of human beings that is medicine.

The history of medicine is often chronicled through major discoveries that change practice: the advent of penicillin or insulin, vaccines, transplants, dialysis, new drugs and procedures that cure or manage illnesses previously beyond our control. As important as these technologies are, the skills to use them properly, often referred to as the art of medicine, have evolved significantly as well.

An Evolving Art

During the past twenty years, a number of major conceptual developments have occurred in that art and, subsequently, in the way it has been taught. These include the focus on social determinants of health, patient-centred medicine, social accountability, and evidence-based medicine.

The first – and the most profound, in my opinion – is the understanding of the determinants of health, as discussed in the previous chapter. This is an intuitively true concept, one that was described as far back as Hippocrates and more clearly in the mid-nineteenth century by Virchow. The 1948 United Nations Universal Declaration of Human Rights included the right to health:

> Everyone has the right to a standard of living adequate for the health and well-being of himself and of his family, including food, clothing, housing and medical care and necessary social services, and the right to security in the event of unemployment, sickness, disability, widowhood, old age or other lack of livelihood in circumstances beyond his control.[3]

It is clear that the role of social factors in health outcomes has long been understood, but it has become a major focus of health study only in the past three decades. Its uptake in mainstream medicine has been slower yet, but in recent years it has become a central component of training and a topic of increasing importance in the profession.

The impetus for this shift in our thinking stems from two major research projects known as the Whitehall studies. They explored the health outcomes of employees in the British civil service, which is based in London's Whitehall district. This might seem an unusual source for

A Healthy Society

our thinking about poverty and health, as people who work in Whitehall are not poor by absolute standards. They are government employees with stable jobs, but they provided useful information nonetheless because the British civil service is an extremely hierarchical organization, with very clear social divides. Led by British epidemiologist Michael Marmot, the Whitehall studies demonstrated that a direct link existed between various illnesses and the employment grade.[4] The higher up you were in the civil service, the less likely you were to suffer from a variety of illnesses.

There have been several theories on how class differences produced the health inequalities in Whitehall. Some have posited stress, job autonomy, or simple differences in income. What is clear from these studies, and hundreds of others since, is that there is a social gradient in health. The lower you are in the hierarchy – whether that hierarchy is financial, institutional, or societal – the worse your health will be. And it is not simply a difference between those at the highest and the lowest levels. The pattern runs all the way up, with each level having significant differences from the one above it. This understanding of the health gradient, though now an accepted tenet of public health, is in fact a complete disruption of our perceptions regarding health and longevity, and a major contribution from Marmot and his colleagues.

The second development is the concept of patient-centred medicine. The rule was once Doctor Knows Best, an attitude that lingers in too many clinics today. The physician asked the questions he considered important, examined his patients, told them what to take to feel better, and sent them on their way. The result: frequent misunderstanding between patients and clinicians, misdiagnoses, prescriptions for treatment that patients were unable or unwilling to complete, and patients allowing responsibility for their health to be the doctor's and not their own.

Today's doctors are trained to FIFE: to think in terms of feelings, ideas, function, and expectations.[5] They explore the patient's feelings about their illness, the fears, concerns, or hopes that have driven them to seek care. They then ask for ideas about the cause of their concern, often a very helpful step as patients may clue in on a diagnosis very quickly, based on their own experience and research. Next, physicians assess the effects of the patient's health concern on their function at work, home, or school. Finally, the expectations for the clinical visit are discussed, allowing doctors to understand the patient's goals rather than assuming they are seeking a particular prescription or other course of action. Once this process is complete and the situation well understood, doctor and patient can work together to find the best course of action, be it medication, referral to a specialist, a follow-up visit, or simply reassurance that the symptoms do not indicate a terrible disease. This method may take a bit longer at first, but as one of the generation of doctors who trained this way, I find it saves a great deal of time and guesswork. I've also noticed that when conflict does arise with a patient, it's usually because I forgot to FIFE and focused too early on my own conclusions. Studies of lawsuits against physicians have reached similar conclusions: people are forgiving of honest mistakes, but they're far less willing to overlook poor communication.[6] The end result of a patient-centred approach is an encounter far more satisfying to patient and clinician, better diagnosis, and much greater likelihood of successful treatment.

One interesting result of this approach is that the definition of success has changed. We now talk about meaningful outcomes. The guiding principle is to do what will most meaningfully improve the patient's quality of life rather than focusing on cure rates, survival times, or adherence to strict guidelines. When we understand what is meaningful to patients and their families, we can know whether to move ahead with a difficult treatment or to spare the expense and discomfort. This humanizing approach, based on what is significant in bettering people's lives rather than an insensitive numerical standard, is an important principle to remember when we discuss political interventions as well as medical.

A related change has been a shift away from the doctor as autocratic captain of the health team, holding all the power and giving orders that must be obeyed without question. More and more, doctors are training and working in interdisciplinary teams, recognizing that each profession brings its own understanding and expertise. This collaborative approach results in better overall care for patients. One example of this is SWITCH (Student Wellness Initiative Toward Community Health), an interdisciplinary student-run clinic in inner-city Saskatoon. SWITCH offers after-hours clinical services and health promotion programming to the community, giving an opportunity for students from medicine, nursing, psychology, social work, pharmacy, nutrition, physical therapy, and more to work together in teams from the beginning of their studies. This sort of collaboration allows for better communication between health providers, resulting in better patient care.

The third important notion is that of social accountability. The practice of medicine, the care of the sick, has at its core compassion and attention to those in need. The profession has also been dominated by social conservatism, economic self-interest, and maintenance of the status quo. The World Health Organization defines the social accountability of faculties of medicine as the obligation to direct their education, research, and service activities toward addressing the priority health concerns of the community, region, and/or nation they have a mandate to serve. These priority health concerns are to be identified jointly by governments, health care organizations, health professionals, and the public.[7]

This means going beyond the work of treating the sick to understanding and addressing why they are ill. The parable of the river is often used to illustrate this approach. Imagine you are standing at the edge of a river. A flailing, drowning child comes floating down toward you. Brave soul that you are, you dive in and rescue it. Before you can dry off and recover, another child appears, so you dive in again and bring her safely to shore. A curious crowd has gathered by now. Another child bobs into sight, and another, and another. People take turns fishing them out. Eventually, someone will ask the pertinent question: Who keeps chucking these kids into the water? And hopefully, someone will head upstream to find out.

A socially accountable health system is one that dedicates resources to where they are truly needed, up- and downstream. It is closely linked to health promotion, prevention of illness, and the social determinants of health. Its design is necessarily complex, as limited resources are available to balance the demands of prevention and care. The more dramatic and tangible interventions – treatments and cures that quickly vanquish illness – receive the most attention. The things that forestall those last-resort interventions are easily neglected in budgets and in our daily lives. On the other hand, no amount of prevention and health promotion will ever eliminate the need for health care. We will always be fishing kids out of the river. This complexity in identifying the priority health concerns and the means to address them is what necessitates the involvement of government, health professionals, administrators, and most importantly, the communities they serve.

The fourth major advance in medical thought, and perhaps the most significant in changing science and practice, is that of evidence-based medicine.[8] This term, coined by Dr. Gordon Guyatt of McMaster University, describes a paradigm shift in medical practice. For centuries, medicine was a highly developed apprenticeship. Doctors studied and practised based on what their predecessors had done, anecdotal evidence, conjecture about how things might work, and in later years the recommendations of pharmaceutical salespeople. Clinical science – particularly its standard-bearer, the randomized controlled trial – has allowed us to evaluate tests and treatments much more rigorously. Today's physicians are expected to have a working knowledge of the analysis of evidence and to remain up-to-date in their field. They are assisted by journals, websites, and other easily accessible tools (such as the phenomenal RxFiles,[9] a Saskatchewan government-supported program that offers unbiased analysis of medications based on cost, efficacy, and safety) to ensure that they have the best of science to assist them.

The analogy of the past practice of medicine and the current practice of politics is striking. Rather than relying on the strongest evidence, political decisions are made based on ideology, popularity in polling, and other sorts of best guesses as to what might work. What is needed is a move to evidence-based policy. Canadian Doctors for Medicare uses a tagline that sums this up very well: "evidence-based, values driven." The evidence is of no use until we know what we're trying to achieve. We need to develop the clearest possible understanding of our goals, our meaningful outcomes. We must then understand the obstacles to reaching them and the actions most likely to have the desired effect. From there, we use the best information and examples available to us and continually examine and improve upon our efforts to build a healthy society.

Just as every person is different – even from him- or herself at another stage in life – every country, province, or city, at any given time in its history, offers differing challenges and opportunities. There is no set of universal policies, but rather a broad range of potential tools to be used at appropriate times. Most political disasters stem from the ideological application of theory in the face of conflicting reality. There is, however, a process for selecting the right tool that can be applied in most situations.

Thinking It Through

To introduce that process, let me return for a moment to the study on health disparity in Saskatoon. This landmark endeavour, which demonstrated the gross health discrepancies between Saskatoon's poorest neighbourhoods and the rest of the city, was only the first step. The creative researchers who conducted the study didn't want to deliver their terrible news without suggesting how to turn the situation around, so they went beyond the collection and interpretation of data to try to discover what could be done. They looked at dozens of countries, from Ireland to Japan, and at the policy changes that had ameliorated poverty and improved health in those contexts. They then published *Health Disparity in Saskatoon: Analysis to Intervention.*[10] This offered forty-six recommendations regarding policy options that were tailored for Saskatchewan and would improve health, from short-term strategies for housing and income stabilization to long-term educational and employment initiatives. Although this study was criticized for failing to focus sufficiently on local strengths, it presented some compelling arguments, and for our purposes it offers an example of how evidence-based policy can be made. This process can be divided into four key steps:

Study: Be it a health problem, a business opportunity, or a gap in educational services, the first step is to understand the extent and character of the situation. If this step is to succeed, we must first understand what our goals are. Knowing that we intend to improve the health of the population by addressing the determinants of health gives us a foundation from which to choose what to study. The authors of *Health Disparity in Saskatoon* identified the growing health concerns in Saskatoon's core neighbourhoods and used the available data to better understand the situation.

Plan: Once we develop an understanding of the problem, the next step is to generate a plan of action. This requires diligence. All options must be considered and weighed in the local context. Historical successes and failures, local values and attitudes, existing resources, and more must be taken into account. Perhaps most importantly, the people who will be affected by any change must be consulted in a meaningful fashion, as they can understand their own situation much better than an outside observer could. They may recognize flaws in plans or come up with better ideas that will work locally. Neglecting this participatory element has been disastrous for any number of well-intentioned programs.

Act: The plan as developed must be properly resourced and put into action. Special care must be taken to understand end-points (when an intervention is finished) or program sustainability (how to support an ongoing intervention). Though perhaps the most straightforward aspect of a program, this is the living test. The plan must be sufficiently flexible to adapt to changing circumstances, misunderstandings, and resistance. When community members and those who apply the policy understand and are committed to the underlying reasons for the change, the problems that arise are more likely to be smoothly managed.

Here, unfortunately, is where the health disparities story stalled. It's a common problem. Whether recommendations emerge from an independent group or are commissioned by the government, they remain just that – suggestions for improvement. Without the political will to follow through, which requires involvement from step one, the evidence languishes unheeded. Governments need to be part of the process from beginning to end, committing to a full understanding of how social determinants of health affect the population and applying the policies that will make a difference.

Fortunately, though their recommendations were not wholly implemented, the researchers and health advocates behind the disparities study continued to push for greater equality. They formed the Saskatoon Poverty Reduction Partnership (with representation from provincial and municipal governments, non-governmental organizations, churches, and academic institutions) and identified seventeen of the original forty-six recommendations that had attained broad community, government, and business support, including measures to improve housing, educational and employment opportunities, and to raise awareness of the social determinants of health. As well as doing the hard work of trying to implement these challenging recommendations across multiple sectors, the partnership is developing an appropriate set of indicators to define and measure meaningful outcomes, which leads us to the final step in the process. In Chapter 5, I will explore the Poverty Costs effort that emerged from this partnership and the ways that it advanced the debate on poverty and health in Saskatchewan.

Reflect: No matter how brilliant the idea or how diligently considered its application, the result may not be what was hoped for. Or it may exceed expectations and require further investment. The key is for the evaluation to be transparent; successes and failures must be clearly examined and communicated. A major challenge of government is to receive proper recognition for what it has done well. The current focus is on failure: governments tend to downplay it as damage control, and the media and the opposition try to expose it. Honest discussion of intention and result, owning one's plans and their results, would lead to greater respect from members of the public, particularly if they are involved in the process from beginning to end.

There is an ongoing need for innovations in measurement so that we can better understand both the underlying situation and the effectiveness of interventions. To again quote Virchow, "Medical statistics will be our standard of measurement; we will weigh life for life and see where the dead lie thicker, among the workers or among the privileged."[11] Understanding the social determinants, their effect on the population, and the means of addressing them will require creativity and dedication on the part of scientists and policy makers. Work is under way on many fronts, in Canada and around the world, to collect data on health inequality along with evidence on the most effective means of making change.

Commitment to an evidence-based policy process that is rigorous and transparent will allow those developments to occur.

One example of this work is the World Health Organization's Commission on Social Determinants of Health, led by Michael Marmot, which outlined a global agenda for health equity through action on the social determinants of health. The comprehensive report, *Closing the Gap in a Generation,* lists three "Principles of Action":

1. Improve the conditions of daily life – the circumstances in which people are born, grow, live, work, and age.
2. Tackle the inequitable distribution of power, money, and resources – the structural drivers of those conditions of daily life – globally, nationally, and locally.
3. Measure the problem, evaluate action, expand the knowledge base, develop a workforce that is trained in the social determinants of health, and raise public awareness about the social determinants of health.[12]

This remarkably far-reaching document goes on to explore each of these areas in detail, citing the relevant evidence and charting the steps for addressing the key health determinants. An excellent example of a framework for evidence-based policy on a global level, it is required reading for anyone with a real interest in a healthier world.

As *Closing the Gap in a Generation* demonstrates, the concept of evidence-based policy combines well with the notion of using the determinants of health as a guide for public policy, be it on a national, provincial, or local level. The determinants themselves – economics, education, environment, and so on – are already the stuff of policy. At every level of government, departments are tasked with handling these issues. What is lacking is a framework from which to measure our success.

Health offers us a particularly compelling means of shifting to more evidence-based policy, as it meets the two essential criteria of being both meaningful and measurable. It is a well-established shared value, one that appeals across the political and socio-economic spectrum. It is also something that we can and do measure extensively. Morbidity, mortality, the incidence and prevalence of specific illnesses, these are things we are counting and have been for decades. Epidemiology, the science that studies the distribution of disease, has advanced so much that we can now predict and evaluate the health impact of a given policy right down to the level of a neighbourhood or even an individual.

Health in All Policies

As well as making us think differently about politics and medicine, the quote from Virchow poses a question about politicians. Do our elected leaders see themselves as the physicians of our society? Do Justin Trudeau, Philippe Couillard, or Rachel Notley see their primary goal as achieving the best health for the Canadians who elected them? If they did, we'd probably see a different approach to governing than we have. When we think of government decisions affecting health, we tend to look at the budgets of the Ministry of Health, which have been famously expanding to 40–50 percent of provincial expenditures. Health ministries aren't really charged with health, per se: their role is to respond to sickness. The reality is that health is already 100 percent of our budget. It's just divided up into different ministries. Decisions made in every ministry – education, labour, environment, justice, transportation, agriculture, and so on – all affect the quality of our lives. What if the staff in those ministries made their decisions guided by questions of best health outcomes?

The best example of that approach so far is something called Health in All Policies, a strategy that more and more administrations around the world – national and local – are using to improve public health by co-ordinating activities throughout the whole of government. Health in All Policies "is an approach to public policies across sectors that systematically takes into account the health and health systems implications of decisions, seeks synergies and avoids harmful health impacts, in order to improve population health and health equity."[13]

In Finland, the idea of Health in All Policies has influenced public policy for some time. During the 1970s, the Finnish government launched one of Europe's earliest Health in All Policies projects, targeting a particularly unhealthy region of the country.[14] Rather than simply urging the community to "eat less, exercise more," Finnish policy makers persuaded local butter, cream, bread, and meat producers to reduce the fat and salt content of their foods while introducing oil seed crops and berry production as alternative (and healthier) ways to earn a living. Combined with healthier school and workplace menus and tough anti-smoking laws, applying a health lens to agricultural, economic, and education policies helped to reduce cardiovascular disease in eighteen- to sixty-five-year-olds by 73 percent.

In Canada, Quebec has been an early Health in All Policies leader. In 2002, it passed its new Public Health Act, giving the Ministry of Health the power to review policy from other ministries to ensure that it does not harm human health.[15] This has resulted in the regular use of health impact assessments to review new legislation.

However, this approach does have a couple of weaknesses in its ability to advance health equity. Some public health measures may improve overall health but can actually worsen disparities between groups, as those who are most able to benefit from, say, a smoking cessation or exercise promotion program may be least in need of help. The second weakness is that the process is often reactive, one that applies to new legislation but doesn't dig into existing policies or programs that may perpetuate health inequities.

At its 2016 Closing the Gap event in Ottawa, the Canadian non-profit organization Upstream partnered with Michael Marmot to release "Health Equity Action Lens" (HEAL), a working paper on how to enhance the equity impact of Health in All Policies. The HEAL approach entails

1. System level health inequities audits identifying the current social gradient in health
2. Analysis of relevant social determinants and health outcomes
3. A toolkit for the identification of available policy levers to affect outcomes
4. Evaluation of the effectiveness of implemented changes on health outcomes.[16]

The key difference between Upstream's HEAL approach and previous efforts is the increased emphasis on identifying and addressing inequities rather than simply trying to improve health overall without considering the distribution of health within society. HEAL also proposes a more proactive way of reviewing existing policies rather than assessing new initiatives. It reorients government to using the best evidence to achieve optimal health outcomes, a societal goal that is both meaningful and measurable.

Human health – physical, mental, and social – is the canary in the coalmine of the health of our society. It is a proxy or shorthand measurement for a host of meaningful variables. Using the social determinants of health to guide our policies and health equity indicators to judge their effectiveness gives us a much-needed yardstick. It allows us to move beyond the "gotcha" politics of personality and the goldfish memory of the news cycle to a long-term strategy for real development.

Health for all, understood in its broadest terms, is an appropriate overarching goal for society. It's what a democracy is for. As in medicine, there is no political panacea, no one-size-fits-all cure for what ails us. There is no prescription for change; there is only a process. We must work out our progress "with trembling hands." Using the best evidence and tools to address what really determines health allows us to move toward our goal. Measuring and communicating the results enables us to evaluate progress and change direction as needed. This is a rational and meaningful approach to public policy. This is how a healthy society is built.

3

THE EXTRA MILE

Early one winter morning, in my last year of family medicine residency, the rattling of my cell phone on my bedside table woke me from a deep sleep. My supervisor, Dr. Laura Davis, was on the line. She was concerned about a patient named Cheryl, whom I'd followed throughout her pregnancy. We'd been up late with her, and she'd delivered just a few hours earlier. From our point of view at least, the delivery had been an easy one: ten minutes of pushing and out came a healthy baby boy. Cheryl had a mild second-degree tear that I repaired under Dr. Davis' tutelage. Things were going well, everyone was in good spirits; Dr. Davis even trotted out the old chestnut about the perineum healing if both sides are in the same room. We examined the newborn. A few minutes later, Cheryl delivered the placenta without incident. A few clots followed it and her uterus seemed quite firm. We congratulated her and stepped out to the nursing station to do the paperwork. Great Apgar score, minimal blood loss: a job well done.

A nurse came out shortly afterward to tell us that Cheryl had lost some more blood. We went back into the room and examined her. After expressing a few clots from a boggy uterus, we decided to start an oxytocin drip. This seemed to do the trick, as the bleeding decreased and her uterus contracted more tightly. Satisfied with this response, we left her in the capable hands of the nurses at about 10:00 p.m. In the parking lot, I let my car warm up while I dusted snow off the windshield. I looked around and smiled at the old buildings and the gently falling snow, warmed by a sense of vocation.

Fifteen minutes later, I was opening my garage door when my phone rang. It was Laura. Cheryl was still bleeding; the oxytocin hadn't worked. I turned around and headed back to the hospital. The nurses had given her another medication to encourage contraction. Despite this, Cheryl's uterus was boggy again; each time her abdomen was massaged, a kidney-basin–full of clots came out. We called for cross-matched blood and consulted obstetrics.

The on-call obstetrician arrived and put me on the spot in the way that only attending specialists can. I fumbled through the story of the evening and Cheryl's past medical history, somehow failing to mention her eight-centimetre uterine fibroid until the very end. Thinking back, I honestly can't recall if we'd already decided that the fibroid was the source of the bleeding or if I realized this only when I saw the look of recognition on the obstetrician's face. In any case, it was obvious to him and he got to work. An intramuscular dose of a more potent drug seemed to stem the bleeding, but we started a transfusion to make up for what had already been lost. The obstetrician said he'd follow Cheryl for the night and sent us home. This time, I made it to bed and fell asleep instantly at one in the morning.

When the rattling phone awoke me at six, I was groggy. I'm a big fan of sleep and am reluctantly brought out of it. Laura said she was on her way to the hospital. Cheryl had continued to bleed through the night despite the obstetrician's best efforts, and they had decided that a hysterectomy was the best course of action. The baby was her second child, and she was in her early thirties, so taking this step was less tragic than it could have been, but still a dramatic turn of events. Laura told me that an obstetrics resident and another gynecologist were joining the obstetrician to assist with the operation and that, though she herself was going in to help out and see Cheryl, there was really no need for me to be there. From my position in my warm bed, this made perfect sense, and I said I'd see her in clinic at nine.

My head hit the pillow and bounced. There was no way I could get to sleep with Cheryl in the operating room. I dressed, shovelled six inches of fresh snow from my garage door, and sped across the river. At the hospital, I checked in with Cheryl and Dr. Davis about the night's events, gave Cheryl some words of encouragement, and then scrubbed in as a less-than-essential third assist. We followed Cheryl on the ward throughout the rest of the day. She needed another transfusion but generally did well and managed to adjust to the thought of the hysterectomy and all the implications thereof.

A version of this story was the first article I published in a medical journal under the same title as this chapter.[1] In the article, I focused on the pillow that couldn't hold my head. There was no essential reason that I had to get up and join the team in the hospital. I'd done my job and it was perfectly reasonable for others to take over. And I wasn't an obsessively dedicated resident. I'm sure there were many times when, viewing my input as irrelevant, I abstained from going the extra mile.

So what was different this time? The dean of our medical school, Dr. William Albritton, used to say, "It's all about relationship." Having seen Cheryl throughout her pregnancy, I'd gotten to know her and care about her on a personal level. That morning in the operating room, I wasn't needed for any practical reason, but it felt right to be there, and it meant a lot to her that I came. Laura Davis also played an important motivating role; I respected her as a mentor and wanted to show her my interest in serving our patient. So, as I recall these events a decade later, the faces and real names, the clinical details, and the professional lessons are as clear as if they occurred last week.

In the article, I talked about how we could find ways to increase the level of relationship, the connection between patients and providers. I do my best to be present for all patients (and now for constituents as an elected representative), but it's so much more meaningful when I've been seeing a patient for years, when I know their family, their life story, their sense of humour, their hopes and disappointments. There are ways, in training and in practice, that clinical interactions can be designed to promote more longitudinal exposure to patients, to establish systems that foster empathy rather than drain it. The conditions can be created to make the extra mile a part of the accepted path rather than an occasional and expensive detour.

In the years since I finished training, the role of health care providers as advocates has been increasingly emphasized.[2] In fact, it's become a defining characteristic on which trainees are judged as they advance to licensed practice. For the most part, this has meant a stress on advocacy within the clinical role: pushing for a patient to, for example, see a physiotherapist, have coverage for medications, or get an MRI or specialist appointment in a timely fashion. The help of someone within the health system to access the supports of that system is very valuable. But when we return to our understanding of the social determinants of health, it's clear that advocacy must go beyond the clinic walls to really improve the lives of patients.

Prescribing Money

When I give food to the poor, they call me a saint. When I ask why they are poor, they call me a communist.

– Dom Helder Camara, *Essential Writings*[3]

I first met Gary Bloch at a family medicine conference in Montreal. He made a lasting impression. He has wild curly hair and comes across as a laid-back, hip urbanite, but he speaks with the passion of a true believer. A couple of years later, like many people across Canada, I started to hear a lot more about him, the Toronto doctor who was prescribing money.[4]

To explain what he means by that, Bloch describes one of his patients, a sixty-year-old man whom we'll call Jim. He had lived outside in a tent all over the country for about thirty years. His family had broken down amidst serious mental health issues. He had also experienced two heart attacks while living rough and had literally crawled to the hospital from the bush to get treatment. When he came to the Toronto shelter clinic where Bloch works, he was very hesitant to seek care, but he had reached a point in his life where he knew that he had to change.

Bloch did the usual medical workup and started him on the appropriate post-heart-attack medications. He then asked Jim what really mattered to him. Jim said that he wanted to break out of the life he was living but didn't know how. He knew he needed to get out of his tent, get housed, and rejoin mainstream society. But there was no way he could do that, in Toronto, on $700 per month provided by the Ontario Works financial assistance.

Bloch realized that, from a traditional clinical point of view, prescribing the medications might seem sufficient, but it would do nothing to deal with Jim's real needs. What Jim wanted, and needed, was a lot more than pills. So Dr. Bloch worked with him to apply for disability coverage, which meant that he would receive over $1,100 a month and escape what Bloch describes as the "get back to work, punitive, harsh, stressful basic welfare system."[5] This amount was a huge relief for Jim. He could pay rent, stay housed, get his health together, eat well, and lead a decent life. He reconnected with his family for the first time in thirty years and found ways to occupy himself that he could manage with his ongoing disability. He started doing volunteer work, teaching others survival bush skills, and he got a dog as a companion.

Bloch describes Jim as initially very tentative, angry, defensive, and difficult. Providers were scared to be alone with him; they found it really difficult to get along with him. Though his life is still not easy, he is now pleasant and joyful, and has developed a trusting relationship with the clinic staff. This change in Jim would never have occurred merely from giving him medications to manage his blood pressure and cholesterol. Obviously, those help as well, but what made the real difference was the increased income. Prescribing money helped him get his life in order, which also made it possible for him to follow the medical treatment.

Like many doctors working with vulnerable populations, Bloch and his colleagues were frustrated. The classic medical interventions they were prescribing weren't helping their patients in the way that they needed. They started to experiment with various ways of getting patients the income they needed to have better outcomes. They held "special diet" clinics, where they filled in forms that allowed people with medical needs to receive extra financial assistance to purchase more or better food. Given the higher rates of diabetes, heart disease, and many other conditions experienced by those living in poverty, they believed that poverty itself should be a sufficient diagnosis to justify this extra funding. Eventually, the Ontario government revised the forms to make it more difficult to obtain this funding.

The group working on these problems took the name Health Providers against Poverty and continued to act as the voice of health care providers working toward poverty eradication. Gary Bloch continued to bring advocacy into his work, developing a clinical tool that would make it easier for clinicians to incorporate thinking about poverty in their practice.[6] Providers who used the tool were instructed to screen, adjust risk, and intervene. This is very similar to how doctors approach various illnesses: we ask the questions or do the tests that identify the disease, use the results of that screening to ascertain the level of risk, and then prescribe treatments as appropriate. The difference is the focus on income; in the screening section of the tool that Bloch created, patients are asked whether they have enough money to pay their expenses to the end of the month. This has been shown to be a sensitive and specific test of material need.[7] If the answer is no, the index of suspicion (which sounds ominous but just means the level of concern and degree of investigation) for a wide range of diseases, from cancer to depression, should be increased. This is a general approach, as there is no strict set of evidence-based guidelines for calculating the degree of concern, as there is for stroke or heart attack risk.

The most important step, of course, is intervention. There is little point in screening for a condition if no treatment is forthcoming. The Ontario tool recommends filing personal income taxes to access supports such as GST/HST credits, child tax benefit, working tax benefit, and more. It also describes how to ensure that senior patients are receiving Old Age Security and Guaranteed Income Supplement, and that those with disabilities are getting all the benefits available to them through the tax system and social assistance. The tool also includes links to all the forms required to follow through with this advice.

The idea caught on, and the poverty clinical tool has now been adapted for application in each province.[8] The St. Michael's Family Medicine clinic in Toronto, where Bloch works, has taken this to a new level, hiring a full-time income assistance worker to help patients work through all their income options, from accessing benefits to seeking employment. Other practice groups are developing tools that assess different determinants of health. A Saskatchewan group is developing an electronic survey tool to assess the social determinants of health at the level of the individual patient, connecting the results to the 211 program, a searchable database of a broad range of social supports.

Turning Virchow Upside Down

In the previous chapter, I described the concept of social accountability, how medicine increasingly defines itself in terms of its duty to meet the health needs of the communities it serves, moving from a doctor-centred to a patient- and community-centred approach. This is part of why advocacy is increasingly being seen, not as some heroic extra mile, but as part of the core business of the profession.

The common objection to this idea, and to asking patients about their social circumstances, is that doctors don't know what to do with the information once they have it. If poverty, homelessness, or lack of education are the major problems, what can the physician do about them? How ethical is it to screen for a condition that you don't know how to treat? A new generation of health care leaders is seeking out ways to overcome this impasse by learning how to treat the underlying conditions, not just the symptoms.

Virchow's famous quote about politics as medicine on a larger scale is often used to exhort decision-makers to recognize their influence on the health of a population and to see their role as being in service of greater health. This is an excellent idea, and if politicians truly did see themselves as the public's physicians, we would have a far better society to show for it.

With the concept of the determinants comes the realization that the care we have tended to emphasize – physicians, pharmacists, hospitals, and surgeries – accounts for at most 25 percent of health outcomes and probably closer to 10 percent.[9] This has prompted physicians like Gary Bloch and his colleagues to question their practice and think differently about the best ways to improve the health of their patients. If politics are medicine on a larger scale, perhaps the inverse is true. Perhaps medicine is politics on a smaller scale.

Whether it's in their choice of location, practice population, or changing their methods, more and more physicians are taking the classic parable of the river to heart. Rather than spending all their time fishing kids out of the water, they want to head upstream and stop them from falling (or being pushed) in the first place. The question is, how do you leverage the front-line presence of the physician to make changes in the causes (or, as Michael Marmot would say, the causes of the causes) of illness?

A recent series of articles from the Social Accountability Working Group of the College of Family Physicians of Canada describes these actions as existing at the micro, meso, and macro levels – affecting individual patients or families, communities, or society as a whole.[10] The personal connection with patients and their stories makes the micro the most natural level for them to act on.

Promise

One example of micro advocacy is the story of Promise. She was twenty when I met her, and she and her partner, Jake, were hilarious. They cracked me up with dry humour at every prenatal visit. I was impressed by the fact that Jake always came with Promise, as I often see only moms. My wife and I had just learned that we were expecting our first baby, so I may have been a little more in tune to the prenatal process than usual, although it has always been one of my favourite parts of practice. Promise's baby was born between Christmas and New Year's, and I was on call for the delivery. It went perfectly. Jake was there, along with other family members. Everyone was joking and smiling, taking selfies with the new baby girl and shedding the odd happy tear. It was one of those deliveries that make you see the late-night holiday hours as a blessing rather than a chore.

So imagine my surprise the next day when the nurse at the ward desk told me in hushed tones that Promise's baby was being apprehended. This oddly chosen word meant a baby would be taken away from her mother. I learned that Promise's file had been flagged because her mother, the baby's grandmother, lived in the same apartment and had a history of drug abuse. Naturally, this is cause for concern and something that should be assessed and addressed. However, to remove a baby from her mother, especially during those crucial early days of maternal bonding, is the wrong response.

I spoke with the family, figured out what the real risk was, and called the social services staff to give my opinion. They don't automatically contact the family physician in such circumstances, so my call was a bit unusual, and because it was the holidays getting someone on the phone who had the authority to make a decision took time. Ultimately, I was able to convince them that Alisha, the newborn, should stay with her mom and that other supports should be put in place to ensure that their living situation was safe. Although things didn't work out between Promise and Jake – he's since left the province – Alisha has remained with her mom and done very well. She's smart and funny, and is succeeding at school. Every time I see them in clinic, I think about what her life would be like if she'd been apprehended at birth rather than staying with her family.

Every doctor I know has dozens of stories like this, of being pulled beyond the purely clinical, pushing the boundaries of the professional role to where the help is real and personal. These are the stories they are most proud of and the interactions they find the most rewarding. The stories also tend to be limited in their scope, one patient at a time, but not a systemic approach. The work of Gary Bloch and colleagues is a great example of work at the micro level and of making that work a regular part of practice rather than an ad hoc response to one touching moment. That group also emphasizes that the point is not simply to change clinical practice. Just as health is far more than health care, improving health through increasing access to income must go far beyond clinical efforts. This has inspired physicians to move outside their traditional roles and start advocating for upstream policy changes that will have a real impact on the health of the people they serve by reducing poverty. If health care providers merely help people to get a few more dollars without asking why they're poor in the first place, or help one family to stay together without working for child welfare reform, we will only continue to see patients with the same problems, over and over. The micro level, the work for the individual patient, is the advocacy gateway drug for higher-level action. The goal is not to get doctors involved in direct poverty reduction for the few individuals whom they are able to see: the goal is to mobilize what we have learned from health care to inform policy and address the social determinants for everyone.

Meeting in the Middle

Patients come from communities: geographic areas, ethnic groups, social classes. Health care providers can simply see them in the context of the clinic, or they can try to understand the experience of the community and engage with making that a health-producing environment. One place to start this is by asking questions about who our patients are. Groups like the folks at St. Michael's in Toronto are collecting demographic information about the income, housing, and food security their patients. This gives them a bigger picture of what problems are recurrent in the community and helps them to respond appropriately. The next step is to discover who in the community is already working on those issues and to find opportunities for partnership. This could mean working with a community garden or community-supported agriculture project so that people can obtain nutritious food, or working with tenants' rights groups to eradicate mould and bedbugs in rental housing, or working with legal professionals to help people with their immigration status or problems with their employment.

California physician Rishi Manchanda, author of *The Upstream Doctors,* proposes that this is really a new category of health care professional, one he calls the "Upstreamist."[11] This new model of clinician has the skills and responsibility to ensure that her clinic or hospital systematically asks about where patients live, work, eat, and play, addresses upstream problems through interventions at patient, clinic, and population levels, and builds partnerships with upstream actors, guided by data and equipped with specific skills for upstream process innovation, performance improvement, advocacy, and policy development. Manchanda and his HealthBegins co-founder Laura Gottlieb hope that 25,000 Upstreamists will exist by 2020.[12] Manchanda explains,

> Armed with data, promising new opportunities, and a combination of common sense and cutting-edge technology, modern-day upstreamists are demonstrating what thought leaders dating back to the days of Hippocrates long envisioned. Health care can be better. All it takes is knowing how to integrate the social and environmental conditions that make us healthy into the daily work of patient care. In fact, it's thrilling

to consider the growing number of upstreamists among us, from people who intuitively know that smart medicine starts upstream to the innovators turning that vision into reality on the front lines of medicine. Together, they're part of a quiet revolution to improve health where it begins.[13]

The late Dr. Aidan Halligan, director of Well North, co-founder of Pathway with Dr. Nigel Hewett, and former deputy chief medical officer for the National Health Service in the United Kingdom, described this phenomenon as upstream medicine. He noted, "Burgeoning almost like a pall of smoke over a collapsing service, upstream medicine populates the space between our accelerating volume-based primary care services and our increasingly complex specialised services, which are becoming more distant from primary care."[14]

Perhaps what we're seeing here, and in countless other instances around the world, is the spontaneous emergence of a new specialty in response to the gap that Halligan mentions, a fascinating blend of primary care and public health that connects one-on-one clinical service with a reimagining of the advocate role. The development of a dedicated specialty in upstream medicine could give us a cohort of physicians with the skills to respond to illness but also to help create the conditions for good health at the level of supports for the individual, greater community well-being, and smarter policy for ideal health outcomes. If politics are seen as medicine on a larger scale, with health as the primary goal, and medicine as the small-scale expression of that politic of health, we could see something very exciting. We could see a new generation of physicians who have in mind the policy and social realms in which their patients exist, a new generation of political leaders who have the health of their constituents foremost in their thoughts, and a healthier society overall as a result.

One example of this Upstreamist training at work is the SWITCH clinic mentioned in Chapter 2. Alongside the direct clinical service, the students host skills nights, assisting high school students with their homework, working with Indigenous elders to connect with traditional culture, or offering skills such as CPR training to help get employment. SWITCH is run by the students themselves, so they also learn the skills of good governance, fundraising, and partnership development with other organizations, such as the CLASSIC student law centre, a similar program run by the college of law.

This advocacy at the meso level – collecting community data, working with local groups to improve health, and teaching the next generation of providers how to see their patients in community – can be extremely powerful. Action at the local level often generates the most tangible results. However, once again, it is difficult to work at the community level without realizing that the decisions made at the provincial or federal level play a big role in determining what's possible locally.

Doctors for Refugee Care

On June 18, 2012, I joined dozens of health care providers and concerned citizens in Saskatoon for the first national day of action against the cuts to the Interim Federal Health (IFH) program, which then offered health coverage to refugees in Canada. Providers in scrubs and lab coats, sporting stethoscopes and placards with slogans, marched in similar demonstrations across the country. I recall being struck at that time by the fact that, fifty years earlier in Saskatoon, doctors had gone on strike to oppose the introduction of universal health insurance. Now here was a movement of physicians and other health professionals taking to the streets to defend universal care for the most vulnerable. One speaker at that day's rally was a medical student who was born in Afghanistan and had fled to Canada as a refugee. She told of her family's struggles in getting to Canada via Iran and of how important the health care and other supports were to them when they arrived.

In 2014, the Federal Court of Canada ruled that the Conservative government's 2012 cuts to health care for refugees were unconstitutional, contravening section 12 of the Charter of Rights and Freedoms, which forbids "cruel and unusual treatment." The court ruling was a victory for refugees and those that work with them, and more generally for compassion and common sense. But it was also a victory for a generation of newly politicized health care providers in Canada who fought to reverse the deplorable change in policy from day one.

Canada has long been known as a safe haven for refugees from around the world. For the past fifty years, they were provided with health services, including coverage for dental care, optometry, and prescription medications. Given that people fleeing violence and oppression often spend long periods in refugee camps that lack readily available medical care, they typically have higher levels of illness. In providing for this vulnerable population, the IFH coverage reflected a kind and wise approach to refugee care of which Canadians were rightly proud. In 2012, however, the federal government, under Minister of Citizenship and Immigration Jason Kenney, made sweeping cuts to the coverage, drastically reducing services for all categories of refugees (though they were eventually reinstated for government-assisted refugees) and completely eliminating health services for certain categories except in cases of public health risk. This meant that a refugee with tuberculosis would receive treatment but not one who had diabetes or who was having a heart attack.

The rationale given for these cuts was that they would make the system fair, improve public health, and decrease costs. It's difficult to imagine something less fair than denying health services to someone who has just escaped oppression and violence. As for protecting public health and saving money, denying people primary care means that they are likely to present in our health care system later and when they are sicker. A sicker patient poses greater risk to those around them (for example, if they have an infectious illness), and treating more severe or worsened conditions is also more expensive.

Proof of the human cost of denying a vulnerable population essential care came quickly, with stories of pregnant women being turned away from receiving prenatal care, cancer patients being denied necessary medications, and children with asthma not having access to their inhalers. Just two years in, the economic impact of this decision was already becoming apparent, with a study from Toronto's Sick Kids Hospital showing a doubling of hospital admissions and a spike in costs for caring for children.[15]

The reaction of the medical community and other health professionals, however, was encouraging. Their opposition was not limited to individual activists, but included official bodies such as the Canadian Medical Association, Canadian College of Family Physicians, Canadian Nurses Association, Canadian Pediatric Society, Canadian Bar Association, Royal College of Physicians and Surgeons, and many others. Doctors for

Refugee Care, founded in response to the IFH cuts, organized the resistance from the medical community. It also took more direct action, occupying Cabinet minister Joe Oliver's Toronto office and interrupting announcements from Conservative ministers across the country with questions on the IFH cuts for several weeks. My wife, Mahli, whose practice consists largely of refugee patients, was the main organizer of the Saskatoon rallies and was the local lead for Doctors for Refugee Care throughout these efforts. The group maintained the pressure, staging national days of action every year for four years.

Along with this public activism, the group of providers that made up Doctors for Refugee Care also used more official channels. They collected stories of patients who were refused necessary care because of the cuts. They also gathered evidence of the health and economic impacts of the cuts, using this material to inform a court challenge that resulted in the Federal Court decision. An appeal of this decision was dropped by the newly elected federal government in 2015, and the IFH program was fully restored.

This was a victory for common sense and compassion. It was also a sign of a new leadership emerging from within the health professions. Health providers are becoming more vocal in advocating for better health services for populations in need.

Evidence-Based, Values Driven

One of the most successful physician-led organizations is Canadian Doctors for Medicare (CDM). This group was founded in 2006 by Toronto-based family physician Danielle Martin, in response to worrying trends in the profession at the time. Dr. Brian Day, Canada's most notorious advocate for private, for-profit health care, had just been chosen as president-elect of the Canadian Medical Association (CMA). Having such a high-profile position filled by someone who was openly antagonistic to universal, publicly funded care mobilized those in the profession who were committed to delivering care based on need, not the ability to pay. When I was with CDM, we used to say that a responsive, sustainable publicly funded healthcare system is the highest expression of Canadians caring for one another.

It also described itself as "evidence-based, values driven," meaning that it sought out the best evidence of what generated high-quality, accessible, and affordable care for all, not just the wealthy few. I was lucky enough to be the CDM board member for Saskatchewan for a decade. This was especially gratifying to me, as Medicare was one of the reasons I went into medicine in the first place. I've always been inspired by the story of how Canadians came together to design a system that cared for everyone regardless of financial situation, and I wanted to be a part of providing that care. As a board member, I was also fortunate to witness how the combination of academic rigour and dedication to just access to care made CDM one of the most credible and respected voices in Canada's health care debate.

During that decade, there was an astounding change in the CMA. With a series of presidents who were openly in favour of user-pay, private care, the CMA gained a reputation for being more concerned with the incomes of doctors than the outcomes of patients. Starting with Jeff Turnbull in 2010, the last several presidents (there's a new one each year) have been pro-Medicare. In fact, they've largely left that debate behind and have shifted the focus to how physicians can advocate for improvements in the public health care system and to addressing the social determinants of health. This has also changed the role of CDM, once seen as an adversary of the CMA, and the two organizations now find themselves working together to propose innovations that will improve health services.

This doesn't mean that all is sunshine, of course, as the for-profit forces are endlessly creative in their efforts. There have been fights against user fees in Quebec and private MRIs in Saskatchewan, and Dr. Day has reared his head again in a case that threatens the existence of Medicare. His Cambie Surgery Centre in Vancouver was audited and shown to have overbilled patients by half a million dollars in just one month.[16] There was also evidence of charging patients and the public system for the same service, a form of double-dipping that is illegal under the Canada Health Act. Instead of conforming to the law and amending his behaviour, Day sued the BC government to permit doctors to set their prices as they chose and to allow private insurance for publicly funded services. If he wins his case, the continued existence of Medicare is threatened. CDM is part of a group of organizations supporting the legal fight and making the case in the court of public opinion that Medicare, though imperfect, should be expanded and improved, not undermined.

Acting Upstream

These efforts are among many examples of successful macro-level advocacy, but they still focus largely on health care. Michael Marmot has spoken about the need for "a social movement, based on evidence, to reduce inequalities in health."[17] Building on the ideas of the first edition of this book, a group of friends came together in 2013 to form Upstream, a growing part of the Canadian version of the movement invoked by Marmot. Upstream is a national, non-partisan, non-profit organization that describes itself as "a movement to create a healthy society through evidence-based people-centred ideas."[18]

When I first started speaking publicly about Upstream, I was a bit sheepish about using the word "movement," worried that it might seem rather grand for such a new start-up. But everywhere in Canada, I found more evidence that the movement was real. In the health field, among those in public policy, and increasingly in the general public, work is under way that demonstrates an appetite for and application of a new approach. And unlike some of the efforts described earlier in this chapter, it is not solely or even primarily led by health care providers. People from all walks of life recognize the value of health as the primary goal of our political decisions and of the social determinants of health as the road map to reach that destination. Upstream is simply the naming and framing of that existing effort.

The work of Upstream breaks into three main parts: think tank, story shop, and community. The think tank brings together experts – academics, front-line workers, and people with lived experience of deficits in the determinants – to supply the evidence regarding which policy changes would have the biggest impact. Being solid in the evidence is essential to the credibility of the group and also to the viability of the programs to follow. But all the facts in the world won't make a difference if they don't also connect with our feelings. That's where the story shop comes in. By working with writers, photographers, animators, and other creative storytellers, Upstream takes the same approach as this book, using stories of real people to illustrate the effect of bad policies and the possibilities of good ones. These stories are then shared as part of specific issue campaigns, such as the Poverty Costs work described in Chapter 5, and online via Facebook and Twitter. By connecting evidence and emotion, head and heart, Upstream can build a community of individuals and organizations, both in person and online, who can bring the social determinants of health into its own conversations and campaigns.

A stream doesn't change the landscape overnight, and neither will Upstream change the political landscape overnight. But the parable of the river is a sticky idea. Once you've heard it, it's difficult to think about health, or any public policy, in the same reactive, downstream way you always have. As these ideas are discussed, as the rinse-and-repeat cycle persists, they will move from the margins to the mainstream. Eventually, we could see parties across the political spectrum talking about how to address the social determinants of health, because it's what people understand and demand. We've seen this starting to happen, with media references to the determinants and the increasingly frequent use of "upstream" as shorthand for early intervention and forethought. Over time, this concept can act as a social vaccine,[19] the kind of good idea that, when integrated into our thinking, protects us against bad ones.

As Rudolf Virchow wrote, "It is the curse of humanity that it learns to tolerate even the most horrible situations by habituation. Physicians are the natural attorneys of the poor, and the social problems should largely be solved by them."[20] This clearly gives greater influence to doctors than is warranted; it is by no means the role of one profession to determine what will improve the lives of those most in need. The advocacy described here is extremely important, but there is always the risk that, because physicians and other health care providers occupy such a privileged position in society, power imbalances will be perpetuated rather than challenged.

But Virchow's remark does shine a light on the fact that doctors see suffering every day and are trained to identify and remedy it. If they remain diligent, they can resist becoming inured to its inevitability. So long as the goal remains real improvement in the circumstances of the people whom they serve, including greater power and autonomy to determine those circumstances, there is much to celebrate in the new approach to health and advocacy. The renewed focus on health for all, led by trusted voices among the people whose work it is to fight illness, bodes well for politics and for broader well-being in Canada.

4

GROWTH AND DEVELOPMENT

Income is perhaps the most important social
determinant of health. Level of income shapes overall
living conditions, affects psychological functioning, and
influences health-related behaviours such as quality of
diet, extent of physical activity, tobacco use, and
excessive alcohol use.

— Juha Mikkonen and Dennis Raphael, *Social
Determinants of Health: The Canadian Facts*[1]

Income from Within

The road to Tevele is red sand and sloppy in the rainy season. The pickup
truck bounces in and out of ruts as we head thirty-some kilometres
from Massinga to this out-of-the-way rural community, located between
the ocean and Mozambique's national highway. I am travelling with
Dr. Gerri Dickson, director of the Centre for Continuing Education in
Health, and two teachers from that institution, Cipriano and Flávia, both
of whom studied in Saskatoon as part of their teacher training.

The Centre for Continuing Education in Health has a long relationship with Tevele. The *núcleo,* a group of leaders selected by the various
surrounding communities, meets regularly with staff and students from
the centre to address the health needs of Tevele. Over the years, they have

isolated malaria and HIV/AIDS as areas of focus and have conducted various public education campaigns and research projects to try to improve prevention and access to treatment.

Núcleo members, many of them quite elderly, walk for miles to attend the meetings. While waiting for those who are late to arrive, we huddle around a fire built in a hollowed-out section of a large tree to take off the morning chill. After tea, a group of keen participants starts a raucous gathering song: "a kama wasiya" (time is running out). It's a classic, well known by the members, and people clap and dance, animating the meeting grounds.

Like the centre, I also have a long relationship with Tevele. On each of my previous visits to Mozambique, I've taken time away from clinical work at the hospital to learn more about working with communities to improve health. The members of the núcleo are now old friends, and each visit feels like a family reunion. In 2007, I spent an extra week in the community, holding clinics and trying to improve my grasp of Xitswa, the local language.

The visitors and núcleo members gather under a large mango tree to start the day's session. The sun comes out and warms us to the point that we leave our jackets in the back of the pickup. Every meeting opens with the national anthem, "Moçambique, Nossa Terra Gloriosa," which is taken very seriously. Everyone stands at attention, looks straight ahead, and sings in a sombre voice. Passersby on the road to town stop and stand until the song is over. This time, halfway through the second chorus, the rain starts anew. This is no drizzle; it's a tropical, soaked-to-the-skin-in-seconds downpour. Given the solemnity of the song, no one can run and seek shelter. We grin and bear it, water pouring down our faces as we finish the final lines of the anthem, and then run into the newly built community development centre to start our meeting. As always, the topic is the health of Tevele, but today we aren't talking about malaria and mosquitoes. We're talking about money.

The most important determinant of health, much more than access to health care, genetics, or culture, is income. As Dennis Raphael states,

> Income is a determinant of health in itself, but it is also a determinant of
> the quality of early life, education, employment and working conditions,

and food security. Income is also a determinant of the quality of housing, the need for a social safety net, the experience of social exclusion, and the experience of unemployment and employment insecurity across the lifespan.[2]

The members of the Tevele núcleo may not have read the latest research on the social determinants of health, but every day they see how income shapes well-being and longevity. Every one of them has lost friends and family members to preventable and treatable diseases such as malaria, HIV, and malnutrition. They see that the poorest families suffer the most, that for the want of a few *meticais,* a child dies at home rather than reaching the hospital for treatment.

One of the younger núcleo members, Senhor Ronaldo, has not been feeling well lately. He has been losing weight and having frequent minor illnesses. His wife had left for South Africa a few years ago, and last year she returned. She died a few months later. Many people from the area go to South Africa for work in the mines and other industries there. Coming home sick from South Africa has become synonymous with AIDS. Ronaldo has worked with the núcleo, educating local communities about HIV/AIDS and other sexually transmitted illnesses. He knows very well that he should be tested and start treatment if he's HIV positive, and he knows that both testing and treatment are free of charge, but despite that knowledge, he still hasn't gone for testing. This is not procrastination: he simply can't afford the fifty meticais (about two dollars) to make the trip in one of the battered Toyota pickups that go regularly to Massinga. If he had some form of income beyond what he can grow on his *machamba* (small farm cultivated by hand), he could get the care he needs. If there were more local income opportunities, perhaps his wife wouldn't have had to leave for South Africa to make money.

Recognizing the importance of local sources of income for their families and their community, the núcleo members embarked on a program of economic development. With the help of Canadian partners and a group of young people called Zambo ni Zambo (Xitswa for "step-by-step"), they started a machamba and a carpentry workshop, and have recently started raising chickens. With help from CIDA (the Canadian

International Development Agency), they built a new "centre of competencies" for meetings regarding the economic projects and storage of related materials. Proceeds from the project go to a common account to continue development, with a portion going to individuals involved, depending on the work they contribute. Zambo ni Zambo also works with another of the centre's partner communities, Basso, on a sewing project and a bakery. The underlying idea is to increase the community's ability to sustain itself economically. This gives local people more access to gainful employment and income for necessities such as travel for hospital care and medications, simple household goods like blankets, and more varied food than what they can grow themselves. It allows them to find this income closer to home, decreasing the disruption to family life and community health brought by migrant work. This goes step-by-step with the health promotion and disease prevention activities of the núcleo, as rather than waiting for help from outside, the people of Tevele start to take charge of their own development. In the long run, these efforts may make a real difference, helping people like Senhor Ronaldo and his family to do better economically and live healthier, longer lives as a result.

Stories like that of Senhor Ronaldo's bring home just how important economic opportunities are for health. From Mozambique to Canada and everywhere in between, economics is the primary practical human activity. The exchange of goods and services governs much of our everyday life. The economic success of individuals has the greatest influence on their health, far above biology, access to health services, or culture. That success is also a significant source of social stature.

I mentioned earlier that health care is always at or near the top of the list of public priorities. Its main opponent in vying for public concern is the economy. People recognize the importance of economic success for physical, mental, and social well-being. The list of health determinants is topped by income and social status, with the position in the economic hierarchy being the single largest factor affecting health. Income also governs many of the other determinants: the ability to afford child care or higher education, safe housing and good nutrition, leisure and exercise, and in many places access to health services. It is little surprise, then, that those at the top of the scale for wealth are there for health as well.

Nor is it surprising that economic success, such a key tool for reaching our goal of health and well-being, can be mistaken for the goal itself. This is a dangerous error. When a tool for reaching our goals is confused with the goal itself, we lose sight of the end and chase the means. Instead of working to improve economies to better our lives, we try simply to improve economies regardless of the effect on people. In this sort of environment, indicators of aggregate success such as GDP growth, rather than finer-tuned tools directed to true well-being, are used to measure our success as a society. And in such an environment, where the inequality of the distribution of ill health and poverty is not considered, a small number of people may become very wealthy and well, whereas a far greater number languish.

For decades, people have decried the inadequacy of aggregate measures such as growth in Gross National Product, or its more commonly used consumption-based cousin Gross Domestic Product (GDP), to assess real progress. Back in 1968, Bobby Kennedy highlighted the flaws of this approach:

> Gross National Product counts air pollution and cigarette advertising, and ambulances to clear our highways of carnage. It counts special locks for our doors and the jails for the people who break them. It counts the destruction of the redwood and the loss of our natural wonder in chaotic sprawl ... Yet the gross national product does not allow for the health of our children, the quality of their education or the joy of their play. It does not include the beauty of our poetry or the strength of our marriages, the intelligence of our public debate or the integrity of our public officials. It measures neither our wit nor our courage, neither our wisdom nor our learning, neither our compassion nor our devotion to our country, it measures everything in short, except that which makes life worthwhile.[3]

Because all growth is lumped together, there is no mechanism to determine whether society as a whole benefits from it. If we look only at monetary transactions, things that cause harm can be seen as positive contributors to the economy. So-called externalities, such as the depletion of finite resources, environmental damage, or offloading of costs to other nations, can be ignored because they have no immediate bearing on monetary transactions. To quote University of Toronto philosopher Joseph Heath, "Anyone who treats economic growth as an overriding policy objective is therefore guilty of committing a 'count the benefits, ignore the costs' fallacy."[4]

The need for a subtler and more sensitive measure of development is acute. The Genuine Progress Index is one such measurement,[5] and excellent work is being done by the Atkinson Foundation on the development of the Canadian Index of Wellbeing (CIW), a much finer instrument for the numerical assessment of various aspects of societal success. The 2014 CIW report showed that despite a 29 percent increase in GDP between 1998 and 2010, the well-being of Canadians improved by only 6 percent during the same period.[6] The 2016 report showed some recovery of both the economy and the CIW after the 2008 financial crash, but the disparity remained with a 10 percent increase in CIW compared with a GDP increase of 38 percent between 1994 and 2014.[7]

Now, if the intended outcome is economic growth, a 38 percent increase in twenty years is a phenomenal success. However, if the goal of public policy is to translate economic activity into the improvement of people's lives, this is a massive failure. If what we're trying to do is practise politics as medicine on a larger scale, it can only be seen as malpractice.

The availability of the CIW and other such measurements of quality of life is a promising change in the way we evaluate the work of governments, allowing us to point to concrete measures and to the specific areas that require attention. However, they have yet to gain real traction among the media and the general public. If we tie them to the natural common interest of health, an outcome that we already measure in great detail, perhaps we can find a way to focus more attention on these efforts.

A Better Pancreas

One of my first public attempts to make the connection between income inequality and health was in 2006 during my family medicine residency.

I was asked to speak to the annual convention of the Saskatchewan New Democratic Party about SWITCH, the Student Wellness Initiative Toward Community Health, as part of a panel that included a young entrepreneur and the publisher of a magazine for Aboriginal youth. The idea was for the party, which then formed the provincial government, to celebrate the successes of young people in Saskatchewan.

At SWITCH, students from medicine, nursing, clinical psychology, social work, physical therapy, pharmacy, nutrition, dentistry, kinesiology, and more work together, under appropriate supervision, to provide after-hours care and health promotion programming in Saskatoon's core neighbourhoods. As well as providing much-needed access to care in this underserved area, SWITCH is an excellent service-learning experience for the students. They learn in a practical, hands-on fashion about the social determinants of health. Perhaps most importantly, they make meaningful connections with real people, taking these key ideas from the theoretical to the personal.

As a student, I worked to establish SWITCH and later spent a year as the project co-ordinator. The Saskatchewan government was generous in supporting the program, coming on early with funding and helping us establish legitimacy as we sought other supports. At the time of the convention, our doors had been open for a year, and I was pleased to share some of the program's successes with our benefactors. I spoke of the hundreds of students on the volunteer rolls, the many different services offered, and the dozens of community members who used those services at each shift.

But I couldn't leave it there, on a falsely positive note. The study on health disparity in Saskatoon, released only a few weeks earlier, gave evidence of growing inequality and the suffering it caused.[8] A condition that we see every day at SWITCH, one that people in the core neighbourhoods are thirteen times more likely to contract, is diabetes mellitus, which occurs when the cells in the pancreas fail to regulate blood sugar. Rather than a proper balance of the fuel that cells need to operate, they have levels that are damagingly high or dangerously low. The analogy to the maldistribution of resources in our society, and the subsequent ill effects on our health, is compelling. Initiatives such as SWITCH and Station 20 West, valuable as they may be, treat the symptoms of a much deeper imbalance. Just as the body needs a mechanism to ensure that the needs of all its parts are met, with no organs starved or overfed, society needs a mechanism to ensure that resources are effectively and equitably circulated. So, tongue-in-cheek, I urged the premier and his party – by enacting policies to more effectively distribute wealth – to become a better pancreas.

Turning the Tide

Aside from the risk of sounding ridiculous, I was cautioned by some against this approach. When applied to wealth, "redistribution" was a dirty word, even among left-of-centre New Democrats. No one talks about that any more, they said. And they were probably right. We talk about growth and the benefits it brings for all, of how a rising tide lifts all boats. But the truth is that, while no one was talking about it, a massive redistribution of wealth had been taking place right under our noses. A small number of people have been apportioned an unprecedented percentage of the wealth in this country. A 2014 report from the Broadbent Institute showed that the majority of Canadians don't approve of this state of affairs.[9] They desire action on inequality, despite underestimating just how unbalanced the distribution actually is. The richest 20 percent now controls over two-thirds of all the wealth in the country, with the poorest 20 percent controlling no share at all.[10] This is the kind of destabilizing growth that undoes development, a disturbing trend for all involved.

In recent years, there has been an overall upward trend in wealth throughout the world. The economies of most nations, with rare exceptions among the poorest countries, are climbing in real terms. You might conclude from this that people's lives, so dependent on material wealth, are getting better. And in many cases, you would be right. Life expectancy is increasing across the board. Indicators of ill health, such as maternal and infant mortality, are steadily dropping.

However, when we look a little closer at the data, a different story emerges. Life expectancy is like the GDP of health indicators; it gives us a sense of aggregate success or failure but can miss pockets of change that go against the grain. Some people are, in relative or absolute terms, getting poorer, and that decrease in wealth is accompanied by an increase in ill health. This is true on the whole in Sub-Saharan Africa and some geographical outliers such as Haiti. It's also true within nearly every nation of the world, particularly the most developed ones known as the G8. The rising tide has not elevated every ship; it has swamped and sunk the smaller craft. Many are left behind or are worse off, despite the overall growth. The whole may or may not be greater than the sum of its parts, but some parts do much better than others. For those who are excluded from economic progress, the result is more sickness and worse health.

It's not only the people in unequal countries that are sicker; it's their markets as well. The OECD reported in 2014 that income inequality is at its highest level in thirty years, with economic growth slowed by as much as 10 percent in some countries as a result.[11] Greater levels of inequality damage the economy, worsening the material conditions of all who participate, and with them their health and well-being.

The province of Saskatchewan, where I live, is no exception on either front. Our overall wealth has increased significantly in recent years. In the mid-2000s, under the government of Premier Lorne Calvert, we went from being a long-standing have-not province – receiving equalization payments from the rest of the country – to being one of the haves. Saskatchewan was booming, and it was touted across Canada as the economy to watch. It was one of the last to suffer downturns in the recession that affected economies around the world. The swelling tide was a source of pride and hope for many.

But not for everyone. My neighbourhood was once known for its low-cost housing. There was lots of rental space, much of it not of particularly good quality, but people could always find a place to stay. Then the boom hit Saskatchewan, and housing prices skyrocketed. Over two years (2006 to 2007), the average price for a house rose by more than 50 percent.[12] There is probably some truth to the observation that this was a market correction of undervalued property, but the shift was dramatic and sustained. Houses were being snapped up for renovation and quick resale, for condos and conversions. Speculation and the home-buying rush pushed vacancy rates to under 1 percent,[13] and rents rose drastically – in some cases doubling in a matter of months. This provoked drastic change in people's lives.

The Little Boats

There's a family that comes frequently to the West Side Community Clinic; we'll call them Lucas and Annie. Hardly a week goes by that I don't see them for a medical visit or just hanging out in the waiting room. They both have chronic medical conditions; he's had some trouble with the law; they've struggled with addictions. They can be friendly and charming, and they can be absolute pains. One of their daughters, Jaelynn, got sick a couple of summers ago. Nothing too serious, but it required some specialist visits and more frequent follow-up with our clinic.

That was the summer we started to see a new kind of homelessness in Saskatoon. The shelters at the YWCA and the Salvation Army were always full. There were more tents in the parks by the river. And in the winter, freezing deaths became a reality, as people slept outside, even when temperatures dropped to 30 or 40 below. In the mornings at West Side, people queued for the waiting room because they needed a place to hang out all day if they weren't welcome in the shelter or at the house where they were couch surfing.

Lucas got picked up for violating his parole conditions and had to spend thirty days behind bars. With him unable to contribute and rent being raised, the family lost their apartment. Annie would get a room for a week at the YWCA, or they'd convince a cousin to let them sleep on the couch for a few days. Despite being hobbled with arthritis, she'd walk for hours with Jaelynn each day in search of an apartment. When Lucas was released, they tried going to his home reserve, but the housing there and in the nearby town was full as well. Despite all this transience, they kept up pretty well with their own medications, didn't use again, and got Jaelynn to all her appointments. She was improving quickly and didn't need any serious treatment. However, after a few months of back-and-forth in temporary housing, Social Services decided that Annie and Lucas were not doing a good enough job of parenting, and Jaelynn was apprehended into foster care.

Aside from the madness of trying to help children out of poverty by taking them away from their parents, this story illustrates an essential point. While the newspapers were talking about Saskatoon's housing boom, many families were going bust. The truth is that when the tide rises, especially if it does so quickly and wildly, the littlest boats get swamped.

This type of story is distressingly common. Economic growth across Canada has not been equally distributed. The gap between the rich and poor continues to widen, with the top 40 percent of earners experiencing real increases in wealth and the bottom 60 percent actually losing income relative to thirty years ago.[14] Canada's income inequality is worsening more quickly than it is in our historically less equal neighbour, the United States. This has happened in Saskatchewan as well, with the wealthiest 10 percent of families earning more than the bottom 50 percent combined.[15] Between 2001 and 2011, the incomes of those in the top 20 percent of Saskatchewan earners rose by seven dollars for each dollar increase among those in the bottom 20 percent.[16] With prices climbing along with wealth, the purchasing power of the average family is falling despite economic growth.

This is not fair. It also costs far too much – in social services, in lost productivity, in lost lives. The question isn't whether we can afford to do something about it. We can't afford not to. The question is, what can be done? How can a government act to change this? It's hard for political leaders, caught up in the glitter of boom times, to put on the brakes. This is especially the case when the prevailing orthodoxy is that since growth is good, more growth, faster growth, is ideal.

Opening the Tool Box

A vocal group of economic thinkers claims that government needs to get out of the way and allow people to pursue their own interests in a rational manner. The invisible hand of the market will sort everything out, and all of us will benefit. It's a pleasant notion, this idea that everyone's lives will improve if people simply follow their own desires. Unfortunately, that is like trying to reach your destination by heading in the opposite direction. People following their own wants cannot meet everyone's needs. Growth, unless deliberately directed, results in the concentration of wealth among the few and increasing poverty among the many. The hand of the marketplace is not only invisible; it is also blind. It needs the guidance of our goals as a society.

Eric Kierans asks, "What can politics do? It must first accept the responsibility of sovereignty and the supremacy of politics in deciding the allocation of resources and the direction of future development. Let the economists decide the application and costs of the directions chosen."[17] We need to change the way we talk and think about the economy. A shift from measuring our societal success by purely economic criteria could allow us to do so. The economy is an essential tool for reaching our goals of full health for all, but it is not the goal itself. Once we realize that, once we put the economy in its proper place as a tool and treat it as neither a force of nature beyond our control nor our ultimate goal, we can start to use it wisely. That opens up all sorts of possibilities.

Economic management has been dominated by two main approaches, laissez-faire versus state involved, with great variation in the degree of each. The former is characterized by minimal taxation and a lack of regulations, the idea being that economies function best when they are unhindered and that external corrections are inherently damaging; somehow, if trade were truly free, if the invisible hand were given full rein, all would be well. The latter assumes that, since the function of the economy is to help us achieve societal goals, society should take control; if we plan and design intelligently, all will be well. It is characterized by subsidies and regulations, often determined less by economic purposes than by political ones, as politicians seek re-election. In such a system, where supply, demand, and consumer choice lose their corrective force, we see stultification of growth and innovation, rampant corruption, and economic decline. As tends to be the case, when we are presented with polar opposites, the truth is somewhere in between. The worst systems have been those in which either approach was taken as dogma.

The principles to preserve here are

- allowing space for innovation and growth (and failure and rebuilding) in a way that encourages entrepreneurship and hard work
- creating a system that is fairly and usefully regulated, enabling citizens and companies to participate confidently in the economy

▶ identifying goals for the economy beyond its own proliferation. This returns us to the notion of meaningful outcomes. Just as in patient care, if we are looking to build a healthy society, we must know what that means.

The economy is not just any tool. It's the principal form of interaction in public life and in much of private life. But it is not that life. The first suit jacket I ever owned was a hand-me-down I wore to my med school interview. It didn't fit me very well and still doesn't. But in the pocket is a piece of paper with a quote from the Renaissance physician Paracelsus that I hoped, and still hope, would guide me in my decisions as a doctor:

> If the physician understands things exactly and sees and recognizes all illnesses in the macrocosm outside man, and if he has a clear idea of man and his whole nature, then and only then is he a physician. Then he may approach the inside of man; then he may examine his urine, take his pulse, and understand where each thing belongs. This would not be possible without profound knowledge of the outer man, who is nothing other than heaven and earth.[18]

Just as we are so much more than the mere workings of our organs, our lives are so much more than the workings of our economy.

To return to the World Health Organization definition of health as full social, mental, and physical well-being, we have a clear description of what our real goals are, our meaningful outcomes. Having understood that health is our goal, we need to ask how we can work with the economy to reach that goal. The economy is a tool to make our lives better. If it fails to do so, we're not using it right. How can we use it more wisely?

The evaluation of any economic strategy (be it intervention or observation) must include not only the question "Will it work?" but also "For what (and whom) will it work?" In what way will it affect the economy, and will that effect be in line with our real goal, a healthy society?

This allows government to take the most important step: to see the economy as a vehicle to reach our goals and economic policy as the tool box that is key to maintaining the vehicle. We must not behave like the proverbial men with hammers, to whom every problem resembles a nail. This is where we get into trouble – when tax cuts or tax increases, privatization or nationalization, become the response to every problem. The appropriate role of government in different industries at different times is one of active intervention or benign neglect. What is needed throughout is not a fixed ideology, but attention and intention, especially in periods of growth. If we understand what we want from our economy, we'll know how to manage it. If we use the tools wisely and appropriately to produce meaningful outcomes for the needs of the time, that management will be effective. If not, the vehicle begins to drive us.

The Case for Fairness: Poverty Costs Too Much

I started this chapter by talking about the impact of income on the other determinants of health. The converse is also true. With a little consideration, it's easy to see how education level, employment conditions, physical environments, and social supports have a great influence on people's income and social status. This is true for individuals, but it also extends to society as a whole. The healthier people are, the better they will perform economically and the better the economy itself will perform. In its 2008 report, "Healthy People, Healthy Performance, Healthy Profits," the Conference Board of Canada outlines the business case for action on the social determinants of health.[19] The report demonstrates how businesses large and small can improve productivity and organizational performance by addressing the determinants for their own employees, can profit by taking the determinants into account when designing and offering products and services that meet pressing needs, and can contribute to the overall stability of the economic environment.

The great thing about efforts to address the social determinants of health by reducing poverty is that, as well as improving people's lives, they also have enormous economic benefits. Poverty itself is a drag on the economy. The Economic Costs of Poverty in the United States study (2007) showed that childhood poverty had a downward effect of 4 percent of GDP on overall economic health.[20] In Canada, poverty is estimated to escalate health care costs by $7.6 billion and result in a loss of $13 billion in income taxes and of over $35 billion in productivity.[21] These enormous costs stem from the fact that when people live in poverty, they are unable to participate fully in public life and the marketplace, and cannot contribute to the tax base. They are also more likely to be involved in criminal activity, which has direct costs (property loss) and downstream costs (lost productivity, prison costs). They also tend to use more publicly funded services such as health services and social assistance programs. A country where fewer people are poor will have a much better functioning internal economy. Business owners will have more customers with more disposable income and a safer, more stable environment in which to work and invest.

This is a neglected aspect of what is needed to have a successful economy over the long term. Investments in physical infrastructure, in roads and other supports that are clearly necessary for businesses to operate, must be accompanied by investments in human infrastructure – in health, education, child care, housing, and nutrition. When we have a healthy, educated populace, able to participate fully in the economy, we all share the benefits. We spend less on social services and enjoy the benefits of enhanced productivity.

When we allow people to fall through the cracks, we all share the costs. This is the functional feedback loop of economic prosperity: at a system level, economic growth improves the health of people, and healthy people improve the economy. At the individual and family level, just as income affects the other determinants of health, they, in turn, have a significant impact on income. The more educated you are, the better your housing, the stronger your social supports, the more able you are to contribute meaningfully to the economy. Where things go wrong is when the system and individual levels don't meet. If some people get healthy and wealthy, whereas others stay sick and poor, fewer people are able to contribute and more require assistance.

Though amassing great wealth has an obvious appeal to those who are able to do so, it has a destabilizing effect on the society that makes them wealthy. Greater differences in income increase social distances. Cuts to health and education lead to heightened social stratification and demand for social services. If these go unheeded as tax bases are eroded, crime rises and is increasingly directed against the wealthiest. If this trend continues, you get political instability that threatens to disrupt the country, including for the wealthy. So, rather than enjoying the benefits of hard work and good fortune, the wealthy find themselves living in gated communities, isolated from and afraid of the dangerous world around them. More equal societies, where the gap in fortunes between those at the top and those at the bottom could feasibly be crossed, are safer and more satisfying to live in.

It's not hard to show people the need for greater equality. They see the effects on individuals and society wrought by economic disparities. Wealthy or poor, many people recognize the stress that such inequality causes in their own lives. The challenge is to find an acceptable means of changing the current situation.

Guiding Growth into Development

> Take the central policy importance given to economic growth: Economic growth is without question important, particularly for poor countries, as it gives the opportunity to provide resources to invest in improvement of the lives of their population. But growth by itself, without appropriate social policies to ensure reasonable fairness in the way benefits are distributed, brings little benefit to health equity.
>
> – Commission on Social Determinants of Health, *Closing the Gap in a Generation*[22]

Economic growth can be an effective tool for improving people's wellbeing. As the story of Senhor Ronaldo illustrates, where economic opportunities are few, as in Tevele or many parts of Canada, growth is exactly what's needed. A more active economy is essential. Though distribution must be a consideration in times of scarcity, it is not nearly as important as finding more resources.

Once a certain level of economic prosperity has been attained, however, there are diminishing returns. When that plateau has been reached, real benefits in terms of outcomes that are meaningful to health and well-being are best produced by better organization in the distribution of the proceeds of growth. Redistribution is far more efficient and effective than economic growth in addressing wealth inequality and the well-being of low-income families. The challenge before us is how to make the transition to development, how to make growth work for us: slow it down, speed it up, or tame it for our real good rather than being pulled blindly along by it.

The pendulum swing between good times and bad, richer and poorer, sickness and health is an accurate description of Canadian history and a potential vision for the future. As a province that has traditionally been dependent on raw material and natural resource industries such as mining, agriculture, fossil fuels, and forestry, Saskatchewan is particularly susceptible to the ebb and flow of world markets. The same can be said for most regions of Canada. If prices for our goods are low, we do badly. If prices are high, we do well. Sometimes, we do spectacularly well.

Boom times are like an illicit drug. They're exhilarating and exciting, but they come with serious side effects. People forget that interest rates went through the roof, farms were forced into foreclosure, and families walked away from their mortgages in oil-rich Calgary in the 1980s. They forget that booms have always been followed by busts and fail to plan for what happens when the downturn comes. The boom is fuelled by policies that foster undifferentiated growth, without a plan for development.

The eventual bust, on the other hand, is often countered with austerity measures. These include cuts to key services such as health and education, privatization of publicly owned companies or lands, and paradoxically, cuts to taxes for corporations and the wealthiest. We saw a textbook example of this in Saskatchewan's 2017 budget.[23] Revenues from oil and potash had dropped considerably, and increases in spending during the preceding years had left the province with growing debt and no reserves. The governing Saskatchewan Party chose to introduce deep cuts to education, eliminate funding for hearing aids and podiatry services, cut the wages of public workers such as teachers, police, and nurses, and shut down the provincial transit service. The only area of the budget that saw a significant increase was in social services, but this was in the total amount, not the individual allocation. This meant that poor people weren't getting any more money, just that the government was expecting to give money to more poor people. They even removed funding for funeral services for people on social assistance, which, given the impact of the rest of their policies, may have been the only long-term thinking in the budget.

Obviously, that last remark is tongue-in-cheek, but the reality is that austerity leads to greater illness, both immediately and in the long term by undermining key services and slowing economic recovery. This has been shown around the world and here in Canada, and is perhaps best illustrated by the concept of fiscal multipliers, or the amount of money returned to the economy in response to a particular policy. Corporate tax cuts tend to have low rates of return, with little to no increase in jobs and a fiscal multiplier of 0.2.[24] In other words, for every dollar you cut in corporate taxes, 20 cents is returned to the economy. In stark contrast, investments in infrastructure, housing, and measures to assist low-income families return $1.30 to $1.50 for each dollar invested. Similar numbers have been reported for investments in health and education, and it makes sense. If you take good care of people, they are able to weather the storm. But responding to a falling economy with austerity measures is like handing an anvil to a struggling swimmer. As economist Nick Falvo wrote in his review of the 2017 Saskatchewan budget, "Good budgeting invests in people while strengthening the economy. This budget did neither."[25]

We will be stuck in this boom-bust cycle of wild spending and drastic cuts unless we recognize the difference between growth and development. Just as a tree farm is not a forest, a quickly growing economy is not necessarily a developed economy. Growth is an essential part of the economy, just as it is an essential part of cells, the building blocks of life. Cells must grow and develop and differentiate. Unchecked growth – growth for its own sake, with no intention and direction – is cancer. Development, on the other hand, is when that growth is applied, serving to improve society and create opportunities for further benefits.

Pediatricians who examine a child aren't satisfied to know that they are advancing along the growth chart, increasing in height, weight, and head circumference. They ask the parents about gross motor skills, such as turning over, crawling, or starting to walk, and fine motor skills such as grasping objects between two fingers. They ask how many words the child knows and whether they understand the world around them through interaction and play. No one would be satisfied if a child simply got bigger without showing some evidence of development; why would we be happy with an economy that grows without being certain what it's growing into? As Kenneth Boulding trenchantly observes, "Anyone who believes in indefinite growth in anything physical, on a physically finite planet, is either mad or an economist."[26]

Positive growth happens when we take the gains from our natural resources and invest them. We invest them in physical infrastructure, to be sure, but more importantly, we must invest in human infrastructure: in education, in health, in housing, in transportation. That will give us a healthy, educated population that can take the gains from boom times and convert them into stability.

We must also consider that booms are generally based on non-renewable resources, things that will eventually run out. The bust may be inevitable; the next boom is not. As a medical student, I visited Uranium City in northern Saskatchewan. Once a thriving community of five thousand, it's a ghost town now. A beautiful high school and crescents of suburbs stand abandoned and vandalized, a monument to short-term thinking. The uranium is gone, and the people with it. Many years may elapse before it comes to this in other industries, but we can't plan our future on things that won't be around forever.

We should plan our future on what will keep. The momentum of boom times should be used to create an economy that, rather than booming and busting, will bloom and last, an economy grounded in long-term sustainable development. The knowledge economy, educating the next generation of scholars, can create an environment for research and innovation. An energy industry based on inexhaustible resources such as sunshine and wind can expand markets, create jobs, and provide for our energy needs. These and other industries based on resources and services that are stable in both demand and supply need to be the backbone of an economy that can weather busts and properly direct the force of booms.

Closing the Loop, and the Garage Sale

In Saskatchewan, we export nearly everything we grow and import nearly everything we eat. We have productive land and a population that is too small to eat everything we grow. But we are able to produce only certain things, so we cannot meet all the needs and wants of residents, meaning that importation and exportation are inevitable. Though trading is an essential part of our economy, however, the current situation is unbalanced. We export things that we could consume and import things that we produce. More pathological perhaps, our economy includes the export of raw materials that go through relatively minor value-added production (logs to boards, wheat to bread, livestock to meat) outside the province and are returned to us. The waste of profit and jobs, and the negative environmental impact of transport make a strong case for closing the production-consumption loop.

Promoting knowledge economies, sustainable development, and value-added production is all part of the move from a garage-sale economy to one based on sound financial planning. No one would suggest that a family should rely on selling their furniture, appliances, and clothes as their sole source of income. Yet this is what we do when we rush to extract resources as quickly as possible. There's no plan for the days when the cupboard is bare. Governments are often exhorted to behave more like businesses. Wise businesses don't sell everything they have and hope for more to arrive. They diversify their investments, take calculated risks, and plan for the future.

A more apt analogy, given the responsibilities and relationships involved, is that of government as a household. Wise families seek out sources of income, managing debt cautiously and investing in the future. They take care of themselves, they feed and clothe their children, and make sure they get the education they need. When something goes wrong, they get help from available services and from social supports, the family and friend networks they maintain. In short, they address the determinants of health; they do what it takes to make their family as healthy as possible. Government should be an extension of this approach, managing the resources and laws at its disposal for the common good and seeking at each turn to choose wisely for the health of the population.

Finding the Balance – Incomes to Outcomes

The most direct, and perhaps the most achievable and measurable, way of addressing the determinants of health is to focus on making incomes more equal. Roughly put, there are two main ways of equalizing wealth. The first is post-taxes (progressive taxation), the second before taxes (increased income parity). Whereas the latter is more attractive, as it requires less "taking away" of earned wealth, both are probably necessary to some degree.

An example of a tool box approach to economic management, one that reaches for the proper tool at the proper time rather than applying a one-size-fits-all approach, is the appropriate use of taxation policy. Taxation levels that impede economic development are unwise. That much is apparent. However, this idea has been taken to ridiculous extremes, with taxes dropping in times of rapid growth for short-term political gain, disrupting public services and costing us money in the long term. What we need is the intelligent embracing of complexity rather than blind adherence to ideology and the approaches of organizations such as the Canadian Taxpayers Foundation, who act as if all collective investment is a bad deal and all taxes are bad taxes (as Prime Minister Stephen Harper famously stated in 2009).[27]

The fact is that most of us save money by paying taxes. When we compare use of public services to income taxes paid, we find that the majority of Canadian families use far more in public services than they pay in taxes. For example, families earning $80,000 a year use approximately $40,000 worth of public services and pay nowhere near that amount in taxes.[28] This is due in part to the progressive nature of our tax system, which charges a higher percentage of tax to those with higher incomes. It is also due to the bulk bin principle; the more you buy, the less it costs. Imagine if each of us needed to pay directly for health care, roads, fire protection, snow clearing – the list goes on and on. Taxes, properly used, are each of us chipping in a small amount to buy something we need at a far better rate than any of us could get alone. The result is a great bargain on things we really need.

A 2014 International Monetary Fund study showed that redistributive policies through tax and transfers not only do no harm to the economy, but can improve performance in the long term.[29] In fact, it appears that public investment in child care and other services is far more effective than corporate or income tax cuts in creating jobs and increasing economic growth.

Those who bemoan any taxation either misunderstand the system or represent the views of the small percentage who pay more than they get back. This, too, is a misunderstanding, as the wealthy, no matter how hard working or intelligent they may be, benefit from public investment as well. This may be directly through subsidies to profitable industries or in the public research and development that is commercialized by companies such as Google and Apple, as described in Mariana Mazzucato's book *The Entrepreneurial State*.[30] On a more basic level, the benefits from public infrastructure, labour, sales markets dependent on the rest of the population, protection from calamity and crime, and access to the natural resources of the land are what allowed for wealth to be accumulated in the first place.

Using this kind of language about collective purchasing power and improved health allows us to talk about taxation in an adult way, rather than getting caught up in false representations that paint taxes as robbing individuals of their wealth and freedom. It opens up space for the discussion of simple changes that increase fairness. For example, in most Canadian provinces, people don't pay taxes on the first several thousand dollars they make. For those whose salaries are small, this is entirely reasonable, but why do people who make a great deal more also benefit from this tax provision? In Newfoundland, the exemption was removed from high-income earners, allowing the lower limit to be increased and eliminating income tax for more people of low income. This helps raise families out of poverty and encourages people to rejoin the workforce, which contributes further to economic growth and decreases government expenditures. This sort of creative means of redistribution through taxation is an effective way of achieving multiple goals: increasing equality, improving health, and contributing to the productivity of the economy.

With all of that said about taxation, however, the truth is that taxes, for historical and psychological reasons, are unpopular. No matter how reasonable they may be, it's difficult for people to get excited about having their money taken away from them. That's one reason to engage in "predistribution" by exploring other strategies for levelling pre-tax income. This can be done in many ways, such as

- expanding training, education, and work entry programs, particularly for people from marginalized groups
- implementing policies to decrease the costs of housing and nutritious food for low-income families
- helping people get off social assistance, not only by ending clawbacks for those who find work, but also by enhancing support during their transition to full employment
- ensuring through indexation that minimum wages are always sufficient to keep working people above the poverty line, thus guaranteeing that a working wage is also a living wage
- protecting or enacting fair labour laws to safeguard people's right to organize and collectively bargain for their wages and working conditions
- and facilitating community economic development, such as the Tevele núcleo or Station 20 West, in communities where stagnant economic growth and lack of jobs are the main barriers to income.

These are just a few ideas for how a wide-open economic tool box, one guided not by ideology but by utility, can help us to move toward our goal of a healthy society. Using health as the measure of success rather than blunt instruments like GDP allows policy makers to adjust wisely in pursuit of that goal.

This is not to say that the economy is not important. Quite the opposite. Income and social status are the factors with the greatest impact on the health of individuals and populations. The economy is too important to be left to dull tools and outdated ideologies. It's too import-ant to be measured badly. Too important a tool for accomplishing our goal as a society to be confused for the goal itself.

As former Saskatchewan premier Lorne Calvert always said, with-out economic progress, social progress is impossible.[31] By the same token, economic progress that erodes the social base on which our prosperity depends cannot be sustained for long. Social progress is economic prog-ress. When we work to build a healthy society, we are also working to build the economy that can sustain and enrich that society.

5

THE SEARCH FOR A CURE
TO POVERTY

Imagine doctors suddenly discover a disease that they'd previously over-looked. Once they recognize it, however, it becomes clear that it is a huge problem. Over 10 percent of Canadians are directly affected: young and old; men, women, and children. It kills more people per year than stroke, diabetes, accidents, and COPD combined. Billions of dollars are lost through decreased national productivity and increased health costs. Flying below the radar of traditional understandings of illness, this disease has quietly been loading an enormous burden onto Canadians.

If a new disease with such disastrous consequences did materialize, certainly there would be a massive outcry. We would expect the government to have a plan in place immediately, mobilizing all the necessary resources to find a cure and prevent the spread. We would demand national campaigns informing citizens of the risks and the quick establishment of treatment centres across the country.

Well, there is a condition that's having exactly this devastating impact right now in Canada. Its name? Poverty.

The negative health impacts of poverty are astounding, making it the most urgent preventable health issue facing the country. People living in poverty are at a higher risk than other Canadians of a broad range of communicable and non-communicable diseases and injuries. The additive effect of all of these conditions is a mortality rate double that of the rest of the population. Forty thousand excess deaths per year have been attributed to poverty; only heart disease and cancer kill more.[1] People living with poverty suffer higher levels of a litany of infirmities: diabetes, COPD, heart disease, depression, HIV/AIDS, and various types of cancers.[2] Over 10 percent of Canadians are poor, and this results in a loss of over $80 billion per year to the national economy through decreased productivity and increased health and social service costs.[3]

Of course, poverty is not new, and no one is suggesting that it was discovered by doctors, but they are paying unprecedented attention to its health effects. A generation of physicians and other health care providers has been trained with an understanding of the social determinants of health. Chief among these is income; how much money we make plays a direct role in our health, and it affects all the other determinants as well. This understanding has led physicians and others interested in health outcomes to start seeing poverty as the major underlying cause of illness. You might think of this in the way we think about diabetes. When you have diabetes, your body can't control the level of sugar in your blood. However, high blood sugar is rarely the direct cause of death or injury. Instead, the elevated sugars harm organs in the body. They damage blood vessels in the eyes, kidneys, heart, and brain, leading to blindness, kidney failure, heart attacks, and strokes. Ignoring high blood sugar and waiting to treat someone's stroke wouldn't make any sense: the mainstay of diabetes treatment is controlling sugar levels to minimize the likelihood of organ damage. Poverty works like diabetes, manifesting itself as other conditions such as heart disease, depression, and cancer. Yet we don't approach it in the same way, choosing instead to treat the resulting illnesses rather than trying to cure poverty itself.

Preventing those complications, and others to follow, means dealing with the root cause, not just the symptoms. As this drive to think – and act – differently in response to sickness develops, more and more people are warming to the idea that we should take what we have learned in addressing health problems and apply it to social problems. If we start to see poverty as the real disease, we can apply the best of our knowledge regarding how to deal with illnesses to the task of developing a truly healthy society.

Too Little Too Late – Lisa's Story

My own connection to this movement stems primarily from my experiences as a medical student, resident, and now a practising family physician. I've had the opportunity to work and to learn in Brazil, India, Mozambique, and the Philippines, all over rural Saskatchewan, including with Indigenous communities in the North, and in my practice at the West Side Community Clinic in inner-city Saskatoon. I consider myself extremely fortunate to have visited and connected with these communities. I've learned to speak new languages, participated in festivals and traditional ceremonies, and found myself welcomed into people's homes. I've shared in lives that were extremely different from my own and have shared some of my life as well. People have generously told me their stories, and I've done my best to learn from them and, where I could, to help them be healthier and happier.

This work has taken me to remarkable places – places I didn't even know I wanted to visit. But sometimes it leads to places I'd never have wanted to be. One such experience stands out in my mind. I have a clear mental image of standing in a cemetery on a reserve in northern Saskatchewan, watching a family I knew well bury their daughter, Lisa, a twenty-five-year-old mother of two. I got to know Lisa and her family during the three years I was her doctor. She had a great sense of humour and made strong connections with everyone on the health care team, though she was sometimes very challenging to work with. Lisa isn't her real name, of course, but she knew that I shared her story. She used to tell people, "Meili's writing a book about me." Most of my patients just call me Meili. They're a friendly, if not overly formal, bunch.

The first time I met Lisa, she came to see me at the clinic in Saskatoon about pain in her back. Two years earlier, she had been struck by a car, which had fractured her pelvis. The subsequent surgery had been successful, but one of the screws that pinned her hip in place had worked itself partway loose. I could feel a piece of hardware sticking out of her back. And so could she; it was a source of constant, unrelenting discomfort.

That same day, I got in touch with the orthopaedic surgeon who had done the original repair to see if it could be fixed. In the meantime, I prescribed something for Lisa's pain. Given its severity, and what she had received in the past, I opted for hydromorphone, or Dilaudid, a derivative of morphine. I gave her a prescription for a week's worth and scheduled a return visit a week later so that I could see how her pain was, follow up with surgery, and find out more about her history and her health.

She came to see me the next week, not exactly when her appointment was, but she showed up. I asked her how things had gone with the medications I'd prescribed. She told me that it helped, but that she hadn't used it as directed. Rather than taking it by mouth, she had injected it. This struck me as remarkable. Not the fact that she'd shot up and misused a prescription; that happens all the time. No matter how careful you are – and my colleagues and I are extremely cautious – some patients will sell or abuse their medications. What amazed me was that she brought it up. I didn't spy track marks on her arms or grill her about her use. She just volunteered the information. I have always taken this as a sign of someone who, for all her difficulties, at the heart of it all, wanted to get better, to be better.

Still, her admission put me in a tricky spot, one that doctors find themselves in quite frequently. Here was a patient with significant pain, clearly in need of treatment, but she was using her pain medication in a way that was too dangerous for me to ignore. So I didn't ignore it, I tried something different. I gave her a prescription for a long-acting opioid, one that the pharmacist can provide daily and observe her taking. This may seem somewhat paternalistic, but it's a regular part of working with people who have serious addictions. The temptation to divert or misuse drugs is so great that, at the very least when first starting treatment, witnessed therapy is an essential tool for making sure what we prescribe goes to the right person in the right way. So that's what we did for Lisa, and she continued to come to clinic and get to know us better.

Unfortunately, one of the things we came to know was that Lisa had contracted HIV, likely from sharing needles when injecting drugs. She'd known she had hepatitis C for a while, but the HIV was a surprise and it sent her into something of a spiral. She started using more, working the street more, and connecting less with us. She was homeless, bouncing from one friend's place to another. Her CD4 count – a measure of the strength of her immune system – dipped down to under a hundred. To fight off infections, it needs to be at least two hundred; most people without HIV have a level of about a thousand. She would show up in clinic when she had pneumonia or another infection but would not come in regularly enough that we could consider starting her on anti-retroviral medications. We knew what to do medically to bring her HIV under control and help prevent these infections, but she had to take pills every day or it wouldn't work.

This went on for a few months, and then something strange happened. One day she noticed a lump in her neck, so she went to the emergency room. A surgeon did a biopsy of the lump, cutting out a small piece and sending it to the lab for analysis. It turned out to be cancer but, oddly, a cancer that isn't associated with HIV. It seemed, as the old saying goes, if Lisa didn't have bad luck she'd have no luck at all. All of the trouble growing up, getting hit by a car, hepatitis C and HIV, and now this.

Strangely enough, however, this cancer may have been one of the best things that happened to her. Somehow, it scared her in a way that HIV did not, maybe because cancer was something she knew she should fear. HIV had become so common in our neighbourhood, where the yearly rate of new cases has been as much as triple the national average, that everyone knew someone living with the disease. Everyone also knew someone who had died from AIDS, as we have very high rates of morbidity and mortality from the illness. In other parts of the country, less than 5 percent of people who have HIV die of AIDS. In Saskatoon at the time, it was over 80 percent.[4] Still, for some reason getting HIV wasn't the shock to Lisa that you'd expect. It was so common that it was normalized. It still upset her, but it didn't drive her to make change. Cancer did. She swore she would fight it, and she did.

That was by no means a straightforward fight. She had to start on her anti-retrovirals to get the HIV well enough controlled that she could handle the further weakening of her immune system from chemotherapy. This wasn't easy, as she continued to struggle with drugs. She got kicked out of the hospital half a dozen times for using. She would disappear just before a key appointment, putting her treatment back by weeks. But she kept coming back, and the team of outreach workers and doctors and nurses kept fighting, advocating for her to have one more chance after one more chance. And, to our great surprise, it worked. She took her meds, got her HIV under control, and managed to complete her chemotherapy. She also connected with her family, seeing her children and her parents more than she had in years. She even moved out of the neighbourhood, getting into supportive housing and away from the worst temptations.

She still slipped once in a while, but it really seemed that she'd turned a corner. She was happier and more together than we'd ever seen her. Then something happened, and no one really knows exactly what. She just started to go downhill. Her cancer was gone and her HIV was well controlled, but she kept losing weight. She wound up in the hospital again, looking weaker than she ever had. The team of doctors ran all kinds of tests but couldn't find what was wrong. It was as if the weight of her misfortunes had become too great to bear. She was transferred to a hospital nearer to where she'd grown up and, one day a week or two later, just stopped breathing.

Lisa's story can seem very clinical, full of references to medications and lab tests, of new symptoms and efforts at treatment. But in reality, it's not a clinical story at all: it's a political story. Lisa wasn't sick with HIV or cancer. She was sick with poverty, with a truncated education from becoming a mother too soon, with never having access to good food and never having had a safe place to stay. She was sick with the abuse she'd suffered as a girl and a young woman, and with the marginalization of First Nations people throughout Canadian history. She was sick with the intergenerational effects of residential schools, with having parents who didn't know how to be parents. She was sick with the addictions that emerged from the substances she used to dull the pain of all these deprivations and mistreatments.

We talk a lot about underserved populations in health care, the people who don't have access to a family doctor or can't see a specialist. Lisa wasn't underserved in that way; she saw more doctors and nurses and support workers in the last two years of her life than most of us ever will or would want to. I'm sure there were times when that treatment wasn't the best – I know she was sometimes dismissed or insulted because of who people thought she was – but she did get a lot of support from health care. The simple fact is that the real causes of her sickness could not be undone. Her life had been broken from the beginning, and all the doctors and hospitals, pharmacies and nurses in the world couldn't change that.

We could point to bad choices, as is so often the reflex in stories like these. Certainly, Lisa didn't always choose the healthiest path for herself. However, how much choice did she really have? Growing up where she did, in poverty and poor housing, in the family circumstances that she did, she had a limited ability to make good decisions, or even to know there were good decisions to be made. The story of her battle with the disease of poverty is indeed a story of bad choices, but those choices were made by bureaucrats in Regina and Ottawa, some long ago, some continuing today. Political decisions determine the distribution of wealth, of access to good food, of affordable housing, of just treatment. When we scrutinize what choices lead to poor health, we need to put these political decisions under the microscope.

Lisa's is a tragic story, and like every tragedy, it is all her own. At the same time, like so many others in Canada, it is the story of people who have grown up in poverty, who have been excluded from society and opportunity. It is the story behind the statistics of health inequalities, of the real people whose lives are represented in early mortality and heightened disability.

We need to offer support to people whose lives are already in these circumstances, but much more importantly, we need to prevent them from winding up in such dire straits in the first place. If we are to improve the lives of people like Lisa – and there are so many like her – we need to think beyond health care. Spending our time treating the symptoms will get us nowhere, because the underlying causes continue unimpeded. We're back to treating the heart attack when we should have been treating the underlying diabetes.

If the causes of sickness are political, then the solutions must be political as well. To truly improve health outcomes, we must address the roots of sickness: unemployment, adverse childhood events, social isolation, homelessness, and food insecurity. In a word, if we want people to be healthy, we need to find a cure for the real disease. We need to find a cure for poverty.

A Stethoscope over the Heart of the Matter

A few years ago, I was asked to teach a class of medical students about poverty and health. The class had been taught by two colleagues of mine, amazing nurses who had a lifetime of experience working with the poor. During their lectures, they poured their hearts out but felt that the students didn't really get it. So I asked myself, with nowhere near the life experience, how do I get them to care about this? How do I speak their language?

During medical school, my perception of my classmates was that a third of them were there for traditional or conservative reasons: money, prestige, a good career. Another third were there for altruistic reasons: they had a vocation to serve and wanted to make the world a better place. The middle third was sympathetic to the social mission of medicine but weren't planning to take any personal risks or rock the boat.

This is obviously an oversimplification, and the new generations of medical students suggest to me that the ratio is changing, with more and more students pursuing the profession out of a sense of social justice. Still, that idea, it helps me to think about who I'm speaking to when I stand up in front of a class. The truly insightful students want to know how my presentation will make them better doctors, how it will change their approach to the next patient. The majority of them may just be asking, will this be on the exam?

In that environment, lectures on broad topics such as poverty or the social determinants of health are a tough sell. When I was a student, I was definitely among the social justice third – that is what drew me to medicine – but I still struggled to stay awake during the lectures on the "soft stuff." Perhaps that had more to do with how much I enjoyed life outside the classroom than with how engaging the content was inside, but you see my point.

So when I sat down to prepare a lecture about poverty, I thought about the way that students learn to learn in medicine. They go from having vague ideas about the workings of the body and the various ways those functions can break down to having a very specific framework for understanding and describing diseases. As their training proceeds, they soon become adept at thinking in categories, dividing illnesses into the rare and the common, the dangerous and the benign, and learning the accepted structure for the description of a disease.

This isn't necessarily a recipe for free and critical thinking, and it can produce the attitude that anything not covered in the *Toronto Notes* medical textbook is not real. On the other hand, it creates a useful template for structured thinking and memorization. Knowing about these frameworks helps us get inside the mind of a doctor as he attempts to describe an illness, and the mind of a medical student as she tries to learn from her senior colleagues.

Knowing this about how medical students think, I came up with what seemed an odd idea at the time. What if, rather than rattling off what my listeners would see as sob stories and statistics, I spoke to them in a language they would understand? So I provocatively titled my lecture "Is Poverty a Disease?" *Merriam-Webster's Dictionary* defines a disease as "a condition of the living body or of one of its parts that impairs normal functioning and is typically manifested by distinguishing signs and symptoms." I posed a challenge to the students: Is it reasonable to think of poverty as such a condition?

Just like a deficiency in an essential nutrient, poverty means not having what you need to be healthy. As I mentioned at the beginning of this chapter, this deprivation results in a laundry list of chronic and acute conditions. At first, labelling poverty a disease appears to be a leap in logic. However, the more I described it as such, the more it became clear that, though poverty isn't what we'd regularly think of as a physical pathology, its effect maps perfectly onto our understanding of illness.

Mapping a Malady

Knowing that medical students are a tough crowd, I tried to make my case in language that would appeal to them. When describing a disease, doctors use a simple structure designed to focus the learner's attention on key details. They start with an overview of the scope of the illness and move to its treatment and the likely outcomes. First, they define the illness and discuss its epidemiology, the way it's distributed in society. This includes facts such as its incidence (number of new cases in a certain period) and prevalence (number of cases overall) in a given population. These statistics provide an idea of the frequency of a condition, as well as the sense of who is most susceptible to acquiring it. It is at this point where we might consider the cost to society – in treatment and lost productivity, for example – of the disease.

This model can be applied to poverty, starting with a definition of what poverty means and its epidemiology. An understanding of who is poor and why helps to ground the discussion in real people. Where in Canada are people poor? What is the breakdown by age, ethnicity, gender? What are the gaps in our knowledge and understanding of poverty?

Alongside the epidemiology, we usually discuss the etiology, or the cause of the disease, and its pathophysiology, or the way it makes us sick. In memorizing the various causes of illness, students often use a mnemonic device (memory aid) – VITAMIN D – which stands for vascular, infectious, traumatic, autoimmune, metabolic, inherited, neoplastic, and drug (toxin). These categories are useful for understanding where a condition fits in, and they can help doctors to arrive at a diagnosis. Some of these same categories are interesting to play with in thinking about the causes of poverty. Is poverty contagious, infecting neighbourhoods and communities? To what degree are poverty and its health effects inherited, passed down in a family over generations?

Largely, however, we need to look at macro-economic policies and local resources as the key causal factors in leading to poverty. The distribution of who is poor in a society helps point us to the policies that result in the dissemination of wealth and opportunity. From there, we would look at the pathophysiology, asking what it is about being poor that makes people sick. The lack of basic material needs for good mental and physical development is an obvious answer, as are toxic levels of stress and the challenges in making health choices.

This leads us to the next step, diagnosis. Once you know the disease you're looking for, how do you decide if someone has it? Here we describe signs and symptoms, and the various tests and measurements that turn clinical suspicion into a definitive diagnosis, and that are useful to monitor decline or improvement.

How do we know if an individual patient is poor? The first way is to ask them, which more and more physicians are starting to do as part of clinical history. Asking about income can be helpful, though the answer can be misleading: how much people make matters less than how much they are obliged to spend in meeting their needs. Asking patients whether they have enough money to make it to the end of the month has been shown to be a sensitive measure of relative poverty. Food security and core housing need are other useful surrogate measures of poverty that can help with diagnosis.

Once the presence of a disease is established, we naturally turn to treatment. When should it begin? What options are available? Which is the most effective, the least damaging to the patient, the least costly? It is here that a fundamental question is also posed: Is the illness a chronic one, for which only supportive treatment is available, or can it be cured?

Many remedies have been applied to poverty. There are maintenance types of treatment, akin to managing a chronic disease such as diabetes with a lifetime regime of oral medications or insulin. Social assistance, or welfare, is a model that gives people a small amount of money each month, not quite enough to meet their needs, but enough to scrape by. Other models include a guaranteed annual income of sufficient funds to live reasonably well, overcoming the so-called welfare wall and creating the potential for an individual or family to thrive. More curative models look at education and employment, the means for people to get out of poverty and stay out, no longer requiring a regular treatment. Beyond the individual, we would also look at system-level methods of redistribution that would remove large numbers of people from poverty, as has been done in many provinces with poverty reduction strategies.

Lastly, there is the question of prevention. Once we know what a disease is and how it affects people, can we ensure that no one catches it in the first place? Whether through vaccines, health promotion, sanitation, or public policy, preventing an illness can be far less costly than dealing with it after it begins, not to mention the avoidance of suffering for patients. How do we identify who is at risk and then move to protect them from becoming ill? If we apply this concept to poverty, how do we create the conditions for fewer people to find themselves in poverty? If we took an evidence-based approach to designing policy, could the disease of poverty become a thing of the past?

An Ailment Has Its Moment

As so often happens, just when you feel you've come up with a novel idea, you discover that others are thinking along the same lines. In researching my talk for medical students, I came across an article authored a few months earlier by Perri Klass, a pediatrician who writes for the *New York Times*. In this piece, titled "Poverty as a Childhood Disease," he urged readers to "think for a moment of poverty as a disease, thwarting growth and development, robbing children of the healthy, happy futures they might otherwise expect."[5]

It appears there is now a growing movement among physicians, public health professionals, and activists for health equity to start thinking in those terms. This includes Dr. Gary Bloch and his group in Toronto, who have used this understanding of income as the primary determinant of the health of their patients and have found ways to prescribe their patients money. Other groups are discovering that the health argument is an effective way to call for more generous social programs. Public health departments are raising the alarm on the health impacts of income inequality.[6] National medical associations are releasing papers on advocacy to address the social determinants of health.[7] What was once a fringe concern has now become a mainstream idea in medicine and is ripe to spread to the rest of Canada.

The notion of poverty as a disease that can be diagnosed, treated, and potentially even cured brings a new paradigm to bear on an age-old problem. Framing the discussion in terms of health enables us to appeal across political and ideological lines to a core Canadian value, opening up a conversation that could allow us to be world leaders in creating a healthy society through shared prosperity.

Poverty reduction strategies have become a part of the Canadian policy landscape in recent years and have been implemented in most provinces. In some, such as Newfoundland and Labrador and Quebec, they have significantly decreased the number of people living in poverty. As of 2014, only Saskatchewan and British Columbia had no poverty reduction strategy. A campaign was launched that year in Saskatchewan as a partnership between Upstream, a local food bank, the Saskatoon Health Region, and the Anti-Poverty Coalition. They called their group Poverty Costs, as this was the main message they wanted to convey: the substantial economic, social, and health costs of poverty. To achieve the goal of convincing the province to adopt a poverty reduction strategy, they used the Upstream model of evidence, story, and community described in Chapter 3.

Poverty Costs started by crunching the numbers, using a methodology pioneered in Ontario to demonstrate that $3.8 billion is lost to the Saskatchewan economy each year.[8] That's 5 percent of the province's GDP. Similar estimates have put the cost of poverty in Canada at upward of $80 billion per year.[9] About two-thirds of this comes from decreased economic activity, as marginalizing 10 percent of the population means diminished consumption and production. The other third comes from the increased health, social services, and justice costs that result from lives led in poverty.

The group worked with people living in poverty to share stories of their experiences – stories like that of Olivia, a young girl whose mother had to quit her job because Olivia needed glasses. That might not make a lot of sense, but her low-wage job didn't pay enough for her to afford the glasses. They were covered if she was on social assistance, so she quit her job to be able to get the glasses her daughter needed. Obviously, that was a step backward for everyone involved – Olivia, her mother, and society as a whole – but many programs are designed in such a way that they make it harder for people to leave poverty.

Poverty Costs then used the $3.8 billion figure and the stories it had gathered to mobilize a public campaign, with thousands of individuals and organizations asking the provincial government to finally commit to a province-wide strategy. This ask had been made many times before, but something in the combination of economic and human cost arguments caught the attention of the public and ultimately the premier's office. In the fall of 2014, Premier Brad Wall announced a commitment to establish a strategy. He went farther, asking members of the Poverty

Costs team to join an advisory group that would write recommendations for what the strategy should contain.

The Advisory Group on Poverty Reduction consisted of five members of the community (of which I was one) and high-level representatives from the Ministries of Education, Social Services, Justice, Economy, and Health. We met over several months, working to develop recommendations for a plan with clear targets and timelines to reduce poverty, and the most evidence-based and practical means of achieving them. We came to a consensus, proposing the ambitious goal of cutting poverty by 50 percent in five years, dropping from the current 10 percent (as calculated by the Market Basket Measure) to 5 percent by the end of 2020.[10] This would be achieved via measures in health, food security, housing, education, and employment, but the most important were in income. Recognizing that income is both the way in which we measure poverty and the primary determinant of many elements of poverty, such as access to housing and the ability to afford food, we selected a bold measure as our first recommendation: a pilot of a basic income guarantee.

Back to Basic

The most direct and simple way to decrease the number of people who can't pay for their basic needs is to give them the necessary money and the supports to use it well. The years since 2012, when the first edition of this book was released, have seen an explosion of interest in the idea of a guaranteed annual income, or basic income guarantee. Simply put, basic income goes beyond traditional models of social assistance. These tend to give people far less than they need to survive and then claw back any extra earnings, trapping people behind a "welfare wall" of ongoing poverty. Basic income takes a different approach, assuming that if people have their basic needs met, they will be free to pursue employment or education or, if those options aren't available, will at least be thriving rather than struggling with ill health and other problems.

This idea is not new, but it has experienced a new life, partly because of research into some old data. During the 1970s, the federal government launched a program in Winnipeg and Dauphin, Manitoba, called

Mincome.[11] Residents who had no income were given a monthly sum that equated to 60 percent of the low-income cut-off. The working poor received a smaller amount, depending on how much money they made. When government priorities changed due to the economic crisis of the late 1970s, the program was cancelled, and its results were not really examined until 2006, when Evelyn Forget, an economist at the University of Manitoba, dug into the data. What she discovered was very interesting. The reflex criticism of this type of program is that it weakens the incentive to work. This did not appear to be the case for Mincome: the only recipients who worked less were mothers who spent more time at home with newborns (there was very little maternity leave in the 1970s) and young men who stayed in school instead of quitting early to work.

Aside from not showing the feared "moral hazard" effects, Mincome resulted in a very positive health impact, with an 8.5 percent drop in hospitalizations among the low-income populations, along with decreases in mental health and general practice visits.[12] According to the Canadian Institute for Health Information, Canadians spent $67.3 billion on hospital services in 2016; in today's environment, an 8.5 percent shrinkage in health spending would result in savings of $5.7 billion.[13] No wonder, then, that this information is fuelling an increased interest in basic income, especially among doctors. The General Council of the Canadian Medical Association passed a motion in support of basic income. In 2015, 194 Ontario physicians wrote to Minister of Health Eric Hoskins (who is also a physician), recommending a trial of basic income in that province.

This interest and advocacy from many quarters, including the Basic Income Canada Network, seem to be having an impact. Ontario has just announced a pilot project in which recipients in the communities of Hamilton, Lindsay, and Thunder Bay will be given $17,000 per year,[14] with a top-up of $6,000 more for people with disabilities. It will be very interesting to see whether the outcomes of this experiment resemble those of Mincome and whether it too will suffer the "trial-and-file" fate or be scaled up to the whole province or picked up by other provinces.

Of course, the big question facing advocates of the basic income is how it will be paid for. Evelyn Forget estimated the cost of implementing Ontario's pilot model nationwide at $15 billion per year.[15] That's a pretty hefty price tag but very small compared to the cost of poverty, at $80 billion a year. Naturally, it's not that simple, as the health and social impacts of poverty accumulate over a lifetime. This fact is an ongoing barrier to upstream investment. Governments may want to make investments that will save money over the long term, but they must also find space in this year's budget for things that won't pay off for a decade.

The increased evidence of a positive return on investment from programs that result in happier, healthier people is leading to further examination of this dilemma and ways to overcome it. One study of fifteen European countries in the 1990s and early 2000s showed that each dollar spent in health and education could return as much as 1.7 times the original investment.[16] By comparison, tax cuts, often cited as key for stimulating growth, actually tend to return less to the economy than is spent. So, along with alleviating the costs, social spending can be a powerful economic stimulus.

In 2016, the J.W. McConnell Family Foundation and Upstream proposed a new approach, asking the Public Sector Accounting Board to allow the amortization of evidence-based social investments to be reflected in public accounts.[17] When a government builds a bridge or a hospital, it's recognized that the benefits of that investment will be spread over decades, so the costs can be spread over that same extended period. This is called amortization, and it is an essential financial tool allowing us to build expensive infrastructure now in order to enjoy its use over the long term.

However, when it comes to social investments, no such option is available. All the costs of a social program are borne in the year they are incurred. The return on that investment could be much larger than the initial investment, but the cost of getting started is prohibitive.

Being able to spread those early intervention investments over the lifetime of the predicted effects would allow governments to take meaningful action on the factors that improve the quality of our lives. It would allow action on the social determinants of our health and well-being now, rather than at some hoped-for moment in the future that may never come. Yet, existing public accounting rules don't permit governments to spread their upstream investments over time – even if they demonstrably save money and improve the quality of life of Canadians.

Changing the public accounting rules to allow for the amortization of certain social investments is a potential antidote to austerity budgeting and short-term thinking. Amortization would be a chance to use financial mechanisms invented for another purpose, not only to build bridges of concrete, but to build bridges to a brighter future. It's one way of funding basic income or other major social investments now but spreading the investment over time so that it can be paid for by the savings and economic benefits it generates.

Cost is not the only objection to basic income, and there are legitimate reasons to approach this option with care. Some people see it as a panacea for every problem and suggest that it should replace all other social programs. But we should always be cautious about any treatment that claims to cure too many things; it's the mark of charlatans. A well-designed basic income program would certainly simplify the complex labyrinth of programs and barriers to their access that people living in poverty currently face. But we still need minimum wages and strong labour laws. We still need a well-designed public health care system that includes coverage of prescription medications. We still need affordable housing and affordable child care. Where public policy principles and economies of scale point to government provision of services, such services should not be left to the free market – even if people have a little more money to bring to market. Basic income is about helping people to afford what they need in life, but a big part of that effort is also making life affordable.

Basic income must also be examined through the lens of opportunity cost, weighing its benefits against other new investments such as drug coverage, dental or vision care, or a national housing strategy that might be forgone in favour of it. On yet another hand, if the political moment is such that basic income is possible and other options are not, we would be wise to explore how to do it well. Some policy changes happen slowly, with incremental movements in public opinion. But every once in a while, an idea that seemed to be outside the realm of possibility quite suddenly gathers momentum. In the last few years, the concept of basic income has moved from the margins to the mainstream. Canada seems to have progressed from the question of if to how. A wise approach to implementation of a basic income guarantee could give us the most significant change to the health of Canadians since the introduction of Medicare.

The other major objection to basic income is that, rather than supporting people in precarious working conditions, it will allow employers to pay staff less and treat them worse, with the cost passed on to the public. This is a valid concern, but it's also one over which governments have influence. By increasing minimum wage and enacting strong labour legislation, governments can ensure that working conditions and compensation are fair, and that basic income does not become a subsidy for those who employ the working poor.

Raising the Wage

During the last few years, the "fight for fifteen" has been a rallying cry, as various groups in labour and civil society have pressured governments to raise the minimum wage. They recognize that it is not fair for full-time workers to live in poverty, a common reality due to the combination of stagnant wages and the increasing numbers of people who make minimum wage.

So far, two Canadian provincial governments are heeding the cry. In June 2016, the Alberta government announced its intention to increase the minimum wage from $11.20 an hour to $15.00 per hour by 2018. Although Alberta has the lowest percentage of workers who earn less than this amount, it is still home to nearly 300,000 people whose wages are so low that they cannot afford the basic necessities of life. Alberta's planned increase to the $15.00 level is a first in Canada and has the potential to be one of the most significant public health interventions in the country this decade. Ontario has now said that it will follow suit, raising its minimum wage from $11.40 per hour to $15.00 in 2019.[18]

The link between low wages and chronic illness has been well established, as has the connection with mental health issues such as anxiety and depression. When it comes to child health, a report looking at US birth data for the last twenty-five years showed an association between increases in minimum wage and birth weight – an important indicator for future health – along with increases in prenatal care and decreases in smoking.[19] Better income through a higher minimum wage means healthier workers and families. Bringing the minimum wage closer to a living wage is a simple way to help low-income Canadians enjoy healthier lives by accessing better housing and more nutritious food, and by participating more fully in their community and the economy.

Alongside the health benefits, there are benefits to the economy. As the living wage movement has demonstrated, paying people enough to make ends meet leads to less employee turnover and its associated costs. It also means more reinvestment in local businesses, as lower-income earners tend to spend their earnings locally.

Difficult economic times have tightened provincial budgets. Increasing the minimum wage can help bend the curve on mounting health care costs. It will also ease the pressure on other social programs, sharing the work of supporting those most in need between the public and private sectors. Alberta and Ontario's leadership on raising the minimum wage is a bold experiment in economic governance that other provinces would do well to follow.

A parallel movement to the fight for a higher minimum wage is the concept of a living wage. This is the idea that businesses can and should choose to pay their employees what they need to live. Many businesses are recognizing that when they treat people well, including paying them enough to meet their needs, they keep employees longer, and those happier and healthier employees are more productive. It's one of those cases where the right thing to do – giving people fair compensation for their work – is also the smart thing to do for a successful business.

Working with the Living Wage YXE group, Upstream has calculated that individuals who work thirty-five hours a week would need to be paid $16.19 an hour if they are to "remain healthy, productive, and support themselves and their families with confidence."[20] It's important to note that living wage differs from minimum wage, as it's optional for employers. Living Wage YXE has been identifying local employers who support this idea and has shared their success stories to encourage others to pay their own staff a living wage. Perhaps in time, the concepts will blend, and minimum wages will be living wages. For the time being, they are complementary elements in ensuring that people receive a healthy paycheque.

The fight for fifteen, the living wage movement, and the push for basic income represent a growing awareness that poverty is not something we need to accept. If we are to see it as an illness, then poverty is preventable, treatable, and even curable. And, given its prevalence and the damage it causes, this should be a major focus of our common efforts to build a healthy society.

6

OUT OF HOUSE AND HOME

One afternoon at the West Side Community Clinic, I was handed a patient chart. On the front was a sticky-note that directed me to Room 5 and included a message from the triaging nurse: "Not doing well at school, mother wondering about Ritalin."

I knock and enter the room to see a slightly pudgy little girl playing with the otoscope. She has short, dark hair and pink rubber boots dripping mud on the exam bed. Her mother sees me enter and hisses at her, "Jessica, sit down!"

Jessica is eight, I learn, and has been struggling at school. She's had to repeat one grade already and is in danger of repeating another. Her teacher says she's distracted in class – sometimes disruptive, sometimes simply uninterested. At a recent parent-teacher interview, she suggested that Jessica may have attention deficit hyperactivity disorder (ADHD) and should be put on Ritalin.

Jessica is the middle child of three. Elaine, her mother, is on social assistance. When her former partner stopped paying child support, she and her daughters were forced to leave the apartment she could no longer afford. They spent time at Mumford House, a Salvation Army shelter for women with children, and moved briefly to the small town where Elaine grew up but returned to the city when her relatives could no longer spare the room. Through these transitions, the girls have changed school three times.

Elaine feels fortunate to have found their current place, a basement suite in Saskatoon's Pleasant Hill neighbourhood, where they've lived for two or three months, but she's worried about whether she'll manage to keep it. The month before, during an early season cold snap, the furnace stopped working. The landlord didn't fix it for three weeks, so the family resorted to a fan blowing over stove burners set at high heat to keep warm. When he finally did get the furnace fixed, he grumbled that if they kept asking for repairs, the rent would have to go up. They are already among the 20 percent of renting families in Canada who spend more than 50 percent of their income on housing.[1] Some landlords provide substandard housing at rates that rise in tandem with social assistance rates, ensuring that housing costs continue to squeeze out any money available for anything else. Rent constricts the food budget, making people choose cheap food of poor nutritional value. It squeezes the utility budget, keeping people colder in winter. It squeezes out other necessities such as a telephone, clothes, and laundry services, never mind a few dollars for recreation or entertainment to amuse and distract from the dull desperation of poverty.

In the examination room, Jessica is a bit of a terror, climbing over everything and interrupting incessantly while I interview her mother. When I talk to her about school, however, she clams up. When I persist with questions about her teachers and classmates, she makes noises and faces, and acts up even more. The question before me is, does she need meds?

Ritalin – or, as it is properly known, methylphenidate – is a stimulant drug that, somewhat paradoxically, works to help speedy kids slow down and concentrate. It can be very helpful in treating kids with ADHD. Jessica's struggles at school are consistent with this problem. Even in the presence of these behaviours – which, according to Elaine, persist at home – I'm reluctant to come to a diagnosis and prescribe a medication. Are Jessica's problems really the result of a neurological condition? Considering all the moving, and all the challenges at home, how could we expect a child to be performing well at school? In a reasonable world, we would try to resolve the problems that Elaine and her family are experiencing before treating the symptoms with a drug. This is easier said than done. Perversely, it is often easier for governments to cover expensive, mind-altering medications than to cover families from the elements.

Hoping to get a better sense of their concerns regarding Jessica's behaviour, I give Elaine some forms that she and Jessica's teacher will complete. I also connect her to the social worker on duty and write to Social Services, advocating for increased help with income and housing costs. These are good things to do, but they rarely have great impact. The system is not particularly flexible; it is designed to give the bare minimum for families to survive in poverty, not to help them get out of it.

A Balanced Diet

That same day, Don Bouvier came to see me at the clinic. He's a talkative fellow; when I see his name on my day-sheet, I know that the appointment will take a little longer than usual. With some people, that can be a bother, but with Don I never mind. He always has an interesting story to share and, despite some big challenges in his life, has a pretty sunny attitude. When Don started coming to see me, he hadn't had a regular family doctor for a while, and his type 2 diabetes was badly out of control. His sugars weren't being controlled with oral medications, and if this didn't improve soon he would need to start injecting insulin. I worked with him on getting a new glucometer to test his sugars, adjusted his pills based on those readings, and discussed changes in diet and exercise that could help control his sugars. I also sent him to a physiotherapist and a dietician to do some more in-depth planning around physical activity and healthy eating.

Following up in clinic, I was pleased to see that his sugars had improved somewhat. He was diligently testing and taking his pills at the right time. Despite all this, his diabetes still wasn't well enough controlled, and he was starting to show signs of kidney problems. Because he was already taking the maximum dose of oral medications, he would need to start giving himself insulin injections if the sugars didn't come down further. Though that's not the end of the world, most patients prefer to avoid it as long as possible. I asked him again about diet and exercise.

As a young man, Don was seriously injured on the job, so he can't work regularly. A single father, he takes care of two teenage sons and a nephew. He does some casual work when he's able but is restricted by his disability. His main source of income is social assistance. His ability to exercise is limited; he walks everywhere he can but can do little else without significant pain. As for nutrition, Don has no trouble telling me what he should and should not eat. He understands the recommendations from the dietician and has tried to make some changes, but this is where he runs into real trouble. In his neighbourhood, healthy foods are hard to find and even harder to afford.

As Saskatoon has grown in recent years, the location of grocery stores has shifted. Most are now in suburban districts and are difficult to access without a vehicle. In Don's neighbourhood, there used to be two full grocery stores; both have now closed. Rumour has it that they were profitable, just not at the level of suburban stores. All that remains are convenience stores and a Giant Tiger discount store that carry some groceries, but these are dominated by packaged and junk food. Fresh produce is limited and expensive, as are whole grain foods and fresh meat. This situation is increasingly common across Canada, and urban areas from which fresh, nutritious foodstuffs have largely disappeared have been referred to as "food deserts" or "food swamps," where fast and packaged foods are plentiful, but fresh meat, vegetables, and grains are nowhere to be found.

As a result of his limited income and the scarcity of good food nearby, serving three growing teenage boys with food that they'll eat while following a strict diabetic diet himself is simply beyond Don's means. He is one of many patients with similar stories. In inner-city neighbourhoods and small towns, and especially in remote communities where the cost of basics such as milk and bread can be astronomical, food insecurity is a concern for thousands of Canadian families. Sometimes the problem is a lack of understanding regarding which foods are healthy and which are harmful, but more often it is a matter of affordability and accessibility. People want to eat right, but they don't want their families to be hungry, and the truth is that on a limited budget, bad food stretches further. In Mozambique, malnourished children show obvious signs of their condition: they are emaciated, all skin and bones and sunken eyes. In Canada, the malnourishment is hidden under a layer of fat. Kids are not getting what they need to be healthy, to grow well, and to prevent illness. Instead, they are fed over-processed empty calories, high in salt and sugar – foods that are cheap, tasty, and harmful.

Hitting Where We Live

The determinants of health largely refer to a person's place in society – for example, their wages relative to national averages, the type of employment they have, the family and friends they can count on. These larger realities are hugely influential on our health, but they are in some ways abstract and less immediate than our actual places, our physical environments. The most immediate of these is the home in which we live. Consider, with that, the places where we work, study, and play, the food we eat, the clothes we wear, the water we drink, and the air we breathe, and you begin to get a picture of the inextricable link between our health and the world around us. This is not a contentious assertion. You'd be hard pressed to find someone who would argue that external conditions have nothing to do with the likelihood of experiencing illness.

Despite both intuitive and scientific evidence that supports the connection between where and how we live and our health, improving these circumstances takes a back seat to other spending priorities, or to tax cuts. In Canada, despite reports from all levels of government on the need for comprehensive housing strategies, these same governments have been backing away from meaningful investments in social housing for decades. The most significant such change was the federal government's decision in the early 1990s to stop building new social housing units. It justified this move by claiming that the private sector would be more efficient and effective at generating housing.

The private sector excels at producing homes for ownership or for high-income rental. Developers are good at this because it is the most lucrative segment of the housing market and because their aim is to make profits for owners and investors. Handing over housing strategy to the private sector in hopes that it will make housing affordable for low-income families is like trying to wash your dishes in the clothes-dryer. It's a useful appliance, but that's not what it's for.

The evidence from the experiment of using the private sector as the primary source of social housing bolsters that skepticism. The number of available units has shrunk through condo conversion and the elimination of older rental properties, and the quality of available and affordable housing stock is deteriorating. This means that, despite stagnant wages, low- and middle-income families are paying more to live in worse places. Those who can't afford to pay find themselves in even worse circumstances. Some couch surf. Others crowd into apartments meant for far fewer people, a condition referred to as relative homelessness. A growing number simply have nowhere to go. In large cities and small towns across the country, shelters are too full to accept everyone in need.

Our values as a society, and the harsh realities of our climate, make a growing homeless population unacceptable to Canadians. Advocacy organizations such as Passion for Action for Homelessness, shelter networks such as the Out of the Cold church basement programs that operate in a number of Canadian cities, anti-poverty coalitions, and others continue to work to raise awareness, pressure policy makers, and fill the gaps where they can. Academics and advocacy groups, such as the Toronto Disaster Relief Committee, have proposed what they call the 1 percent solution.[2] Prior to the 1990s, provincial, federal, and municipal governments spent, on average, 1 percent of their budgets on housing. These groups suggest that a return to this level, properly applied with amplified investment in social housing, increased rent supplements for low-income families, supportive housing for those in need, grants for improvement of existing housing stock, and when necessary, temporary shelters for homeless people, could make the Canadian housing crisis far less damaging to people and the economies that support them. Across the country, recognition of the need for change continues to grow, and the demand for a national housing strategy gets louder all the time.

Instead of heeding that cry, governments have shifted from housing strategies to homelessness strategies. Rather than trying to get people into stable homes, they fixate on getting them into short-term shelter. Aside from not delivering what people really need, short-term shelter can cost five to ten times as much as long-term housing.[3] This after-the-fact approach is analogous to concentrating spending on health care rather than disease prevention, where cleaning up the mess costs governments far more than preventing it. It's like a family that decides to eat at restaurants because groceries cost too much. Doing the math shows that a lot more is saved by up-front expenditures; a bit of foresight can save a great deal of expense down the line. Our governments are increasingly reacting, not planning, renting, not owning, and as a result, costing themselves out of all kinds of essential services. Their decision to live hand-to-mouth rather than plan ahead results in worse outcomes for more money. If our friends and neighbours acted that way, we'd shake our heads and think their priorities were confused. Why do we countenance this kind of behaviour from those who manage our taxes?

Taking the First Step

That said, you have to start somewhere. In emergency rooms and frontline clinics, patients are triaged based on the urgency of their illness. The sickest are seen first, followed by those in less immediate danger. A high-quality health system would connect these efforts to a larger plan to prevent illness and keep people healthy but would still provide help in a hurry when things go wrong.

According to the National Shelter Study,[4] Canada's emergency shelters are packed to the rafters. People are languishing in homelessness longer, and their ranks increasingly include seniors, veterans, and families with children. Shamefully, Indigenous Canadians are over ten times more likely than non-Indigenous people to end up in an emergency shelter.[5] In the summer of 2015, the Saskatoon Housing Initiatives Partnership performed a "point-in-time" count of the people who lacked a home on a certain night.[6] It discovered that 405 people were homeless that night in Saskatoon. The number from these counts has steadily risen. In 2008, similar surveys found 260 homeless people, and a count in 2012 yielded 379. Disturbingly, 45 of the homeless in 2015 were children. The sad reality is that more than 35,000 Canadians are homeless on a given night and that more than 235,000 experience homelessness at some point every year, whether they sleep in shelters, on the street, couch surf, or wait unnecessarily in hospital or other temporary accommodation.[7]

Beyond a crisis of housing and poverty, homelessness is a public health emergency. The longer people are without a home, the worse their health becomes. A 2007 Wellesley Institute study showed that homeless people in Toronto were twenty-nine times more likely to have hepatitis C than the general population, twenty times more likely to have epilepsy, and twice as likely to have diabetes.[8] These conditions are related to an interplay between the social and personal factors leading to homelessness and the hardships of living in inadequate housing. Lack of shelter means exposure not only to the elements, with risk of heat stroke in summer and hypothermia in winter, but also to violence. Obtaining safe food and clean water becomes a challenge, and healthy social and family dynamics all but impossible. Managing mental health issues, addictions, and other illnesses is next to impossible without a stable living situation. As a result, hospitalization for unmanaged chronic conditions goes up, as do ambulance pickups to handle emergencies. Cumulatively, these challenges have an untold impact on individuals and a cost of over $7 billion per year to the Canadian economy.[9] A 2014 report from British Columbia suggests that the life expectancy of homeless British Columbians is half that of other residents in the province.[10] These data have led some physicians, such as Toronto doctor Naheed Dosani, to describe homelessness as a palliative diagnosis. All Canadians deserve safe, decent, and affordable housing, but for some, its lack is a matter of life and death. To make the difficult choices ahead, the government should take a page from medicine and triage.

During the last twenty years, as Canada's population has grown, federal funding for affordable housing has dropped more than 46 percent. This means that at least 100,000 units of affordable housing were not built.[11] Canada's homelessness crisis is the direct result of Ottawa's withdrawal from housing investment. In 2015, the new federal government promised a national housing strategy and has embarked on consultations. According to the minister responsible, Jean-Yves Duclos, "the Government of Canada believes that all Canadians deserve access to housing that meets their needs and that they can afford."[12]

Solving all of Canada's housing problems at once, from homelessness to the rising cost of homeownership, would be wonderful. It is absolutely the right objective, but the sheer scale of the challenge when set against political and fiscal realities will force the government to make some difficult choices – something that Canada Mortgage and Housing Corporation president and CEO Evan Siddall acknowledged in media interviews.[13] But the most pressing problem – finding stable housing for those who are currently homeless or at risk for homelessness – can be solved. Housing First is an approach to homelessness that started in the United States during the late 1990s.[14] In the past, the approach to people who were homeless and struggling with addictions or mental illness was "get your life together and then you can have housing." Housing First reverses that notion by recognizing that a stable place to stay is an important factor in getting anyone's life together, whether that means having an address for applying for benefits or work, a regular place to keep and take medications, or just safety from the elements and the violence of life on the street.

A growing number of Canadian cities have been applying the Housing First model, offering housing and direct support to those who struggle the most to find accommodation. A recent study of Regina's Housing First program estimated that housing twenty-six people saved nearly $2 million due to decreases in emergency room visits and arrests.[15] The southern Alberta city of Medicine Hat claims to have "ended homelessness" with this approach, housing more than a thousand people in two years, with shelters seeing occasional brief stays rather than chronic use.[16] As Medicine Hat's mayor, Ted Clugston, explains, "Housing First puts everything on its head. It used to be, 'You want a home, get off the drugs or deal with your mental health issues.' If you're addicted to drugs, it's going to be pretty hard to get off them, if you're sleeping under a park bench."[17]

If we build on these successful examples by linking Housing First with the collection of real-time, person-specific data on homelessness to enable better co-ordination in local planning, targeted investment in affordable rental housing, and a national housing benefit, homelessness in Canada could be rare, brief, and non-recurring. Not only would this take care of those who are most in need, it would free up funds to address elements of our housing challenges that lie farther upstream. The cost savings from shelters and emergency rooms could later be applied to the next steps of providing more affordable social housing, preventing more people from falling into homelessness.

On a system level, public investment in affordable housing has many advantages. Job creation at various skill levels occurs near the communities with the highest unemployment. Although initial investments are required, public money is soon recovered in health, justice, and social services. By shifting people from homelessness to renting, from renting to owning, and from social assistance to employment, a comprehensive housing strategy can decrease costs and increase tax revenues. It can also present opportunities to use what we learn about planning and design to create safe, inclusive, sustainable communities.

Appetite for Change

Lessening the percentage of monthly income spent on housing also helps to address food insecurity, the inability of people to reliably obtain the food they need to live healthy, active lives.[18] In fact, a difference of $100 in rent can decrease food security by over 20 percent.[19] This is vitally important, as food insecurity is a growing issue in Canada. In 2012, over 3 million Canadians – 12 percent of the population – experienced this problem,[20] an increase of 600,000 since 2007. Indigenous families like that of Don Bouvier are more than twice as likely than non-Indigenous Canadians to find themselves in this situation.[21]

The health impacts of food insecurity include difficulty managing chronic conditions, as in Don's case. Growing up hungry can also contribute to various mental and physical ailments that persist into adulthood or manifest themselves there. Along with the obvious cost for the individual, this costs the rest of society as well. A study in Ontario by University of Toronto professor Val Tarasuk and her research team showed that the health care system spent nearly four thousand dollars per year on the treatment of people who were severely food insecure, more than double the cost of caring for people with regular access to good food.[22]

Tarasuk points out, "food insecurity is actually an even better measure of material deprivation than income is. By the time somebody is struggling to put food on the table for themselves and their family, what we're capturing is the product of their income, their assets, their savings, their expenditures, and their debt."[23] Programs are needed that address not only access to affordable food but also the poverty that makes access difficult.

There are local efforts across Canada to deal with food insecurity, including CHEP Good Food in Saskatoon.[24] Starting out as a school meal program, this nutrition-oriented, community-based organization now manages multiple community gardens and collective kitchens in the inner city, helping people to produce and prepare healthy food. It also runs the Good Food Box, a bulk-buying and distribution program that makes fruit, vegetables, and grains, many purchased from local producers, regularly available at reduced prices. These programs are models of the ways in which an approach to food security needs to involve links between agriculture, food distribution systems, education, and economic development.

By themselves, however, community based-organizations cannot meet the need. Community gardens and other programs simply cannot be scaled up to satisfy everyone's food requirements. There is an important role here for corporate social responsibility, with commodity, wholesale, and retail food marketers needing to play their part in ensuring that their services are available to everyone, even if their profit margins are less than those in bigger cities and wealthier neighbourhoods. Where companies are unable or unwilling to provide services, all levels of government must put the proper incentives and regulations in place to make good-quality food accessible and affordable for everyone.

Stories of the inconsistency in Canadian food pricing are well known, with references to ten-dollar quarts of milk and thirty-dollar cabbages in Nunavut a frequent feature. A study of food costs in Saskatchewan showed that people in the Far North paid over twice as much for food than residents of Saskatoon or Regina.[25] This prompts people to ask why a case of beer costs the same in every Saskatchewan town, but food prices vary so widely. These pricing disparities absolutely need attention, but interestingly, the patterns of food insecurity are consistent throughout the country. People with good incomes are not food insecure, even in Nunavut: poverty is the biggest factor that determines who will be hungry and who will not.

Ultimately, food security is more a matter of how income, not food, is distributed. For example, when Newfoundland and Labrador improved social assistance, with higher rates and decreased clawbacks, as part of its poverty reduction strategy, food insecurity among social assistance recipients dropped from 60 percent to 33 percent. This understanding has led many in the food security research community to explore the idea of basic income. In Canada, we have a living example of the impact of this approach, with the Guaranteed Income Supplement (GIS) for seniors. A study of older adults living in poverty showed that their chances of being food insecure dropped by half when they turned sixty-five and started to receive the GIS. Expanding basic income beyond seniors to the rest of the population may be a very effective way of decreasing hunger and the health and financial costs that follow.

To get our house in order as a society and achieve the best possible health outcomes, we need to address the basic needs for food and shelter more equitably. Simply put, this means using the best evidence on what works to ensure that everyone can afford safe places to live and good food to eat. This is the foundation of a healthy nation.

7

THE WARMING WORLD

In 2010, my wife, Mahli, and I spent a few weeks working and teaching in the Philippines. This was an exploratory trip, looking into potential new sites for medical student training at the University of Saskatchewan as part of a program called Making the Links. We were based in Iloilo province in the Western Visayas region and spent some time in the small town of Janiuay (pronounced "Honey, why?"). While teaching the Canadian and Philippine nursing students, we assisted in patient care at the rural health unit, seeing patients in clinic and helping with deliveries. This clinic provides immunizations, medical consults, and obstetrical services free of charge to the general population. This fact is significant, as health services, including in government hospitals and clinics, are too expensive for people to afford. This was a striking contrast not only to Canadian health care, but also to our experience in Mozambique, where the health services were very limited but were all public. If a patient could get to the clinic or hospital, he or she received the care that was available, regardless of ability to pay. In Janiuay, it was quite different, as most of the care was private, including in hospitals.

One afternoon, Mahli was caring for a ten-month-old girl who was severely dehydrated and should have been admitted to the hospital. We accompanied her to emergency, where she was refused care because the family couldn't pay. Staff at the rural health unit told us that cases of diarrheal and gastrointestinal diseases like hers had spiked in recent years. Janiuay had been hit hard by the high winds and flooding from Typhoon

Frank, and many of the poorer people in the community had lost their homes and been displaced. Makeshift accommodations had been set up, but they lacked access to clean water, and the contamination was making people sick.

On the trip back to Iloilo City from Janiuay, I found myself staring out the window, mind wandering as I watched the signs and buildings go by and listening to the students as they chatted cheerfully and occasionally broke into song. I started to think about how the social determinants of health were playing out in the lives of the patients we'd just seen. Due to climate change, typhoons and other extreme weather events are becoming more common, causing injury and death, as well as long-term precarity. People who live in poverty are at greater risk to begin with, and the damage hits them hardest. That little sick baby was the living evidence of the cycle of vulnerability and the way that political decisions put innocent people in harm's way. It was on that trip that I scribbled the outline for the first edition of this book, and over the next two years I gathered the stories and ideas that eventually formed the finished product.

It's notable that an ecological element was present in the story that inspired the original book. No serious discussion of how we view our society can ignore the growing concerns about human damage to the ecosystems that support all life. Discourse on the determinants of health has tended to focus more on the impact of the immediate environments, while ignoring larger concepts of sustainable living. Though the focus on the immediate impacts of individual circumstances is important, it's also clear that air and water quality, climate change, and consumption of limited resources significantly affect our health. We are creatures of our environment, and our health is greatly determined by the air we breathe, the plants and animals we eat, the water we drink, and our ability to live without fear of natural disasters.

In her book *Doughnut Economics*, British economist Kate Raworth uses a circular diagram to depict a safe and just economy as existing in a sweet spot between the social foundation of the determinants of health and the ecological limits of what our planet can provide.[1] It's a powerful image, as it describes a new approach to economies that, rather than pursuing growth for its own sake, attempts to find the balance that would provide the prosperity needed to meet our needs without exceeding the natural boundaries of the planet.

In recent years, the ecological determinants of health have attracted increasing attention. In 2015, Dr. Trevor Hancock led the development of "Global Change and Public Health," a discussion paper for the Canadian Public Health Association that describes the essential "goods and services" provided by the environment on which human life depends.[2] These include the obvious constants, such as the air, water, and food that we all directly consume. They also encompass natural resources and ecological processes such as the ozone layer that protects us from UV radiation, the nitrogen and phosphorus cycles that circulate the nutrients required to grow food, the detoxification of waste products, and the presence of abundant fertile soil, fresh water, and marine aquatic systems to grow food and plants. For humans to thrive, there are three further necessities: materials to construct our shelters and tools, abundant sources of energy, and a reasonably stable global climate with temperatures in the range that can support a civilization. These natural systems form the foundation upon which all other determinants rely and from which they emerge.

Given this, it becomes clear why the World Health Organization has recognized climate change as the biggest health threat of the twenty-first century.[3] The last few years in Western Canada have offered stark examples of the effects of climate change on local environments. Severe weather events and extreme temperatures are increasingly common. Organisms such as the ticks that spread Lyme disease are now establishing themselves in new areas. Forest fires and floods chase people from their homes. Simultaneous flooding and droughts threaten the safety and availability of potable water, and prevent farmers from seeding or harvesting crops. Over time, this volatility can impede our capacity to predict weather cycles for food production, and with that the ability of people to make a living in agriculture.

Climate change is no longer a suspected diagnosis. It's a health emergency that is already causing systemic damage to people around the world. We have made incredible advances in public health and health outcomes over the last few decades, but human actions are threatening this progress.

It's Hot in the Poor Places Tonight

Although the frequency and intensity of environmental catastrophes have increased in recent years, in Canada they have caused comparatively little direct harm to humans. That certainly has not been the case in other countries. As a young man, I travelled to South America to learn what life was like in the lower income countries. I was hosted for the first few weeks at the Saskatoon Roman Catholic diocese mission in União dos Palmares, in the northeastern Brazilian state of Alagoas. Brazil is one of the world's most striking examples of income inequality, a land known for astoundingly wealthy gated communities that overlook sprawling slum cities, or *favelas*. What is seen locally in the large cities of the south plays out geographically as well, with the northeast the poorest part of South America's economic giant. There, the incomes and health status of most people are similar to those in Sub-Saharan Africa. With their crumbling colonial Portuguese architecture and large populations descended from the slave trade, Brazil and Mozambique share striking similarities.

One major difference is in agriculture. Whereas Mozambicans largely rely on subsistence farming, agriculture in Brazil is far more industrial. The northeast is one of the world's largest providers of sugar. Almost all of its agricultural land is used for this purpose, and a large percentage of the population works in factories or cutting cane. Much of the product goes to the Coca-Cola Company, which has significant interests in the area. A small number of *latifundários,* or large landowners, controls the vast majority of land, having over centuries forced most small farmers into feudal service in the cane fields (in Brazil, 1 percent of landowners own nearly half the arable land).[4] Fruit orchards and forests have been converted en masse to sugar cane, causing major changes in local ecosystems.

The town of União is located on the river Mundaú in the shadow of the famous Serra da Barriga (Belly Mountain). The Serra was the seat of government for Zumbi dos Palmares, the leader of a slave revolt that overthrew the Portuguese and ruled the region for nearly a hundred years during the seventeenth century. Each year, pilgrims gather in the historic town, march across the bridge that spans the river, and make the long trek up the mountain in a celebration of resistance and a call for justice.

In May and June, the rains are always heavy, but in 2010 they came heavier than usual. With almost all the land deforested for cattle and cane, the water poured out of the hills in torrents. The Mundaú had flooded before, and people who lived in the streets by the river knew the risk, but it had never been like this. Entire towns in its path were demolished. Water crushed homes, churches, and hospitals. Although some advance warning kept the immediate casualties down, a few dozen people were swept away, and many more were seriously injured, overwhelming what local health facilities remained standing. In the medium term, hundreds of families were left homeless, crowded into refugee camps plagued with water-borne illnesses and mini-epidemics of respiratory infections. Afterward, many flood victims faced an uncertain future: unable to return home to rebuild and unsure of whether the flood relief donations would be enough to establish a new community. Disruption in schooling, food shortages, unstable housing, unemployment, and tragic family losses will affect the health of an entire generation.

This tragedy was compounded by the fact that it was completely avoidable. Organizations such as Movimento Sem Terra (the landless farmers' movement) have spent decades advocating for land reform and sustainable farming practices in the region. Successive governments have promised change, but the forces resisting agrarian reform are powerful. More responsible land use could have prevented, or at least minimized, the flooding. In a more equitable society, fewer people would be forced to live on the marginal riverbank land. And if flooding did occur, there would be more resilience in personal resources and social safety nets, as we see with similar events in Canada.

Perhaps no other industry is so intimately linked with ecology as agriculture. The way in which we farm, be it through choices of transport methods, pest and weed control, or simply location and intensity, has huge implications for soil quality, erosion, climate change, and water safety. The role of the farmer as producer and steward of the land is imbued with enormous importance for the health of all; policy decisions made through a health lens would necessarily involve helping producers to choose methods that are both economically and environmentally sustainable. They would also explore macro-level changes – around fossil fuel use, climate change, and commodity markets – that affect the environment in which farmers operate.

A Fevered Planet

Canada is one of the world's largest contributors to greenhouse gases, with Saskatchewan the highest per capita contributor in the country.[5] Certain aspects of our environment partially account for this: cold winters and long travel distances translate to high energy use, and fossil-fuel-intensive industries such as mining, oil, and agriculture contribute to emissions. That may explain some of our unequal impact on the environment, but it doesn't excuse it. We benefit greatly from the use of non-renewable resources and the associated production of carbon and other pollutants. With the prosperity purchased through that production comes a responsibility to do things differently. The river metaphor comes to life in the Mundaú in Brazil, the Souris in southern Saskatchewan, the raging Red in Manitoba.

The downstream effects of global warming are detrimental to human health at home and abroad. Fortunately, Canada is also in a position (physically and fiscally, and perhaps now politically) to do something upstream. We are blessed with enormous resources in wind, sun, and geothermal energy. We can do some of the forward thinking and investing required to save resources and energy, thus lessening our impact on the wider environment. Though investing in conservation and converting to renewable energy have up-front expenditures, the long-term savings in energy use and health costs make these measures more than worthwhile. If we take action soon enough, there is potential for significant job creation in growth industries related to renewable energy. If our goal is the creation of a healthy population for generations to come, we would be foolish not to shift to practices that prevent damage to the ecosystems that support us.

Canadian Climate Refugees

A young child presents to emergency in respiratory distress, his asthma worsened by smoke exposure. An Indigenous elder has uncontrolled blood pressure because there wasn't time to get her medications when the evacuation orders came through. Scabies and other illnesses related to crowding spread quickly through the close quarters of the evacuees. Sudden departure from and worry about home bring significant mental stress. These sorts of health problems are commonplace for the more than thirteen thousand residents who were forced to leave their homes in northern Saskatchewan due to unprecedented forest fires in 2015. As we look beyond their symptoms to seek for root causes, the connection is fairly obvious: through smoke and relocation, the fires have hurt their health. And the cause of the fires? High temperatures and dry conditions, with climate change the likely culprit.

The people who were relocated in Saskatchewan come from northern communities, where poverty rates are higher than in the rest of the province. This is the predicted pattern of climate change: whether in Brazil or the Philippines, in the prairies or on the coast, remote communities with less infrastructure are more prone to its effects. Poverty, lower rates of employment, the impact of colonization, and other social determinants also lead to higher rates of illness. It also means that community members are more susceptible to the health effects of fluctuations in temperature, air quality, and diet that come with disruption of climate. Although they did benefit from state protection, the internally displaced people in Saskatchewan were as vulnerable as resettled refugees or even more so.

Natural disasters can bring out the best in our political leaders, who come forward with extraordinary support for people affected or displaced by floods or forest fires. We saw this in the Saskatchewan fires and those of Fort McMurray the following year, as provincial and federal governments assisted evacuees and provided additional resources to fight the fires. This action is admirable, a manifestation of the care we supply for each other as a society, and of governments and civil society acting decisively in the public interest.

But paradoxically, tragic times can also be a boon for politicians. They offer a chance to make dramatic speeches and show up at fire stations for photo-ops. This is not to cast doubt on the motivations of politicians. A strong performance at such times demonstrates the dedication that the public expects from elected representatives. However, we should be able to expect more.

To talk about climate change in relation to these events is not merely to bring up politics in a time of tragedy. Politics are already at play. What we need from our leaders is more than a robust response to the downstream effects of climate change. For the health of Canadians, we need to see upstream thinking to prevent this from occurring over and over. Unfortunately, in the case of the northern Saskatchewan fires, we heard nothing of the sort. Much was said about what was being done to help evacuees, but when it came to causes, and specifically to climate change: crickets. We are seeing increasing leadership on this file at many levels, but Brad Wall and the Sask Party have been openly resistant to taking any meaningful action to reduce carbon emissions, even though Saskatchewan leads the country in per capita carbon output.

A Price on Pollution

The flipside of crisis is opportunity. In fact, the central conclusion of the *Lancet*'s 2015 Commission on Health and Climate Change is that tackling climate change may be the biggest health opportunity of our time. This report fused the knowledge of some of the world's most prominent economists, physicians, urban planners, and other experts. Their assessment was that "the single most powerful strategic instrument to inoculate human health against the risks of climate change would be for governments to introduce strong and sustained carbon pricing."[6] The opportunity in question is not only a chance to reduce the health impacts of catastrophic climate change. We are also being given a chance to build a fairer, cleaner, better world.

The *Lancet* likened carbon pricing to methods already used successfully by public health departments across the world, such as tobacco taxation. When the price of something goes up, its use goes down, and market measures are among the most useful means of effecting change. Citing the *Lancet*, the Canadian Medical Association passed a motion in 2015 that committed it to promoting the health benefits of a strong, predictable price on carbon emissions.[7] In 2016, the Government of

Canada announced that it would introduce a national price on emissions in two years. Any revenue gathered through pricing would remain with the provinces, which could design the program as they chose. However, the price would have to apply to all emissions and be equivalent to ten dollars per tonne in 2018 and rise to fifty dollars per tonne by 2022.[8] There is room for the provinces to each choose the best way to introduce emissions pricing, in a way that is sensitive to local realities, and to decide how to use the revenue generated. Conducting a health impact assessment at the provincial level while individual policies are being considered would help ensure that new pricing regimes optimize overall health. In the process, there are some key principles to consider. A fair carbon-pricing system must

> Reduce carbon emissions. There's not much point if such measures are not sufficiently robust to achieve the necessary reduction.
> Employ workers. Ambitious reductions in emissions give tremendous opportunities for employment in renewable energy production, transit, and efficient retrofitting and building, as described in the One Million Climate Jobs plan from the Green Economy Network.[9]
> Protect lower-income families from increased costs. This can be done in various ways. Six of every ten Albertans receive direct rebates to offset any costs,[10] and the majority of them receive more than they spend on the Alberta carbon levy.
> Support producers. Modern agriculture uses high levels of fossil fuels in producing the food we eat. It also results in significant sequestration of carbon through the photosynthesis of the plants grown. A successful carbon price will incentivize more fossil-fuel-efficient farm practices while allowing farmers to keep more of the wealth that comes from their land.
> Protect trade-exposed industries. If other jurisdictions don't have carbon pricing, Canadian industries may find themselves at a competitive disadvantage. A system can be put in place to support them while also giving them an incentive to quickly reduce their emissions.

▶ Speed the transition to the energy infrastructure of the future. Whether through the use of funds gathered through the tax system or simply via the decreased cost associated with producing energy through new methods, carbon pricing must move us quickly to non-fossil-fuel forms of energy production.

Climate change is the biggest threat to human health, which means that a robust response is our greatest opportunity to make positive change. The institution of carbon pricing is a key step in the treatment that will keep us – and our children – alive and thriving.

The Better Story

Climate change is such a massive and complex issue that it can be difficult for people to grasp. As a result, it's also hard to motivate political leaders to take real action in combatting it. Most people can't relate to degrees of warming or parts per million of harmful particles. But humans are hardwired to connect with personal stories. Sometimes what it takes to understand something on this scale is seeing how climate change affects the health of a single person or a community. We can all feel for a young mother, as she watches her four-year-old daughter choking in the emergency room because wildfire smoke is playing havoc with her asthma. As Katherine Burke, deputy director of Stanford University's Center for Innovation in Global Health, states, "I really think that health can put a human face on climate change and can engage our leaders and the public in a much more personal way."[11] A health lens can be a powerful tool for talking about an issue that people are afraid to discuss or find too broad to comprehend. That's why talking about climate change in a way that connects to our fundamental shared desire for good health shows such promise.

The story we currently appear to be writing is a fatalistic account of collective inaction, of short-term self-interest with long-term ill effects. We can tell a better story, one of hope, of leadership, of possibility, of a cleaner future with greater prosperity. We can design a common project that will inspire and excite people. Environmental impact is the most upstream of policy considerations, one that intersects with every other policy area. Balancing the various determinants requires moving beyond simple dichotomies of jobs versus trees to making the complex and challenging decisions to ensure long-term environmental and economic sustainability. Human health can give us a guiding principle through which to make these choices, doing our best to enact the policies that create the conditions for optimal health.

8

THE EQUALITY OF MERCY

Down by Law

During my first year of practice, working at the West Side Community Clinic in Saskatoon, I met a young man whose story has come to represent for me the problems with the justice system. Normally, I would change his name and some details to protect his privacy, but Brad Peequaquat was brave enough to share his story with the *Saskatoon StarPhoenix*.[1] When I first met Brad, he had only recently had an extensive, disfiguring surgery to remove a cancer of the penis. This was radical treatment, necessary to save his life, at least temporarily, from a quickly spreading cancer. Had it been caught earlier, he might not have needed such a surgery and his hope of long-term survival would have been much higher.

The problem is, it was caught earlier. Brad had seen his family doctor when the cancer was a small but worrying lesion on his foreskin. He was sent to a urologist and an appointment was made for a circumcision, a benign and usually curative procedure if done early enough. Unfortunately, through no fault of his own, he never kept the appointment.

Brad grew up in a family with a father who was violently abusive and who regularly committed break-ins and other property crimes. Shown little else in the way of options, Brad and his brothers followed suit, robbing liquor stores and bars, and selling the proceeds in inner-city Saskatoon. This brought him to the attention of the Indian Posse, a gang based out of Winnipeg, and he became one of its local leaders in Saskatoon. Like most members of the gang, he was in and out of prison on various charges.

Unlike most of those young men, however, Brad had a change of heart. He met a woman he cared about, his wife, Joanne, and decided to leave the gang life in favour of fatherhood. He got involved with Str8Up, an organization run by Catholic priest André Poilièvre that has helped more than four hundred young men and women leave gang life in Saskatchewan. Brad and his brothers followed the Str8Up program and found the strength to leave the gang for good. Things were really turning around for Brad, but in 2007 he was caught drinking in violation of his parole and was sentenced to a month in prison.

This is where things went really wrong. Brad showed the prison staff the letter regarding his appointment for surgery. Everything was arranged for him to be taken from jail to the hospital for the circumcision. However, this was a tense time in the corrections system, with a recent high-profile escape, and the guards appear to have been exercising more than their usual control over prisoners. Brad phoned his surgeon's office to talk about his condition, which violated prison policy. In retribution, staff chose not to give him an escort, so his surgery date came and went. By the time he was released and saw the surgeon again, the cancer had spread locally and to distant lymph nodes. A circumcision would no longer suffice; radical surgery was needed, causing significant disability and pain, with little hope of long-term survival. In May 2011, after a long and painful struggle, Brad passed away, leaving behind his wife and a young family.

Brad's story is a monumental tragedy. It is also a glaring example of a justice system that is designed to punish rather than to prevent and protect. This is analogous to a medical system that is curative rather than preventative. The results are the same: more expense, less effect. The people who need help, whether with a medical problem or criminal behaviour, are met too late to make real change. How much easier, and more effective, is it to keep people from starting smoking than getting them to stop? How much wiser is it to keep people out of jail than to try to rehabilitate them once they're inside?

A Healthy Society

Determining Detention

> The degree of civilization in a society can be judged by
> entering its prisons.
>
> – Attributed to Fyodor Dostoevsky, *The House of the Dead*

The same factors that determine one's health determine one's likelihood of coming into contact with the justice system. In Canadian jails, inmates are overwhelmingly of low socio-economic status and have low levels of formal education.[2] They are also disproportionately Indigenous: 20 percent of Canada's prison population consists of Indigenous people, who comprise only 3 percent of the general public. In Saskatchewan, the ratio is even more skewed: 10 percent of the provincial population is Indigenous, whereas a staggering 57 percent of prison inmates come from this background.[3] The same factors that lead to ill health – poverty, lack of education, social exclusion, racial discrimination, unemployment – also lead to imprisonment.

If we want to improve health outcomes, we need to attack the root causes of illness. Similarly, if we want to decrease crime, we need to address its root causes as well. Fortunately, they are the same in both instances. The justice system isn't usually cited as a major health determinant (the numbers of incarcerated people are too small for it to have the statistical impact of the determinants to which everyone is exposed). Nonetheless, incarceration has a substantial impact on health status.

Another way of looking at this is to see involvement in the justice system as a companion indicator of social health: the determinants of health are the determinants of involvement in criminal behaviour. Rising or falling crime rates are clear indicators of whether or not we have produced a safe society, not through intimidation and deterrence, but through an appropriate distribution of opportunity and the common wealth. This is important to consider when designing policy responses to make Canada a safer country: Are more prisons and tougher sentences the right answer? It depends on what you're trying to achieve.

There are three potential reasons to punish someone. The first is retribution: exacting repayment for damage done. The second is risk management: protecting others from the actions of those who do not respect the law. The third is rehabilitation: correcting the behaviour and teaching offenders a better way. In our private lives, in our own homes and families, we discourage revenge as a motivator. Most of us can remember hearing a parent admonishing a squabbling child, "I don't care who started it, you have to stop it." Though it is tempting to hit back at someone who has hurt us, we can easily see that doing so merely perpetuates conflict and justifies aggression. Is it not odd, then, that our judicial system, thought to represent the balanced wisdom of the best legal minds, focuses almost entirely on retribution? There is very little in the way of crime prevention and not nearly enough rehabilitation.

One shocking move away from rehabilitation was the 2009 closure of the farms connected to prisons in cities like Kingston, Ontario, and Prince Albert, Saskatchewan.[4] These farms provided food for the prisons and taught skills to the inmates. Although inmates might not be destined to farm once on the outside, showing up for work, applying themselves to the task, and feeling the satisfaction of a day's labour translate to invaluable experience that can be applied to a return to normal life in society. It often seems that, instead of giving people psychological help or training them in work skills applicable to the outside world, the current system would rather have them sit aimless in jail.

We saw this attitude in action in 2016, when prisoners at the Regina Correctional Centre complained about the food they were being served. Food services at the facility had been privatized. After 115 inmates refused to eat the food, citing raw eggs and other inedible items, Premier Brad Wall said that if they didn't like the menu they should stay out of jail.[5] Aside from displaying ignorance about why people end up in prison, this dismissal of the well-being of inmates showed an ignorance of what is needed to escape a life of crime.

With such an approach, one that ignores the social determinants that influenced the original offence and that are needed to avoid re-offending, inmates may return to life in society exactly where they left off, having just paused for a few years to reflect. More commonly, however, they return worse than they came in, either because they lost ground by going to jail, were physically and psychologically traumatized while there, or had become further involved in criminality through drug and gang activity. Most convicts have little waiting for them on the outside: nowhere to stay, few prospects for employment, and minimal social support. Returning unskilled and undesirable to general society is a recipe for desperation. Add to this the environment in which the last years have been spent, in the company of other criminals, in a culture of gangs, drugs, and violence, and repeat offence becomes even more predictable. Hence the common description of prisons as supplying not correction but higher education in criminality. To return to the health analogy, one could even compare criminal behaviour to a hospital-acquired infection: for the susceptible, there is nowhere as dangerous to full recovery as an institution populated by the unwell, be it a hospital or a prison.

This makes the present emphasis in Canada on increased sentences and the expansion of prisons all the more disturbing. It reflects a further abandonment of prevention and an approach to crime like that which has developed in the United States. In recent decades, American prison populations have skyrocketed, with over 2 million people currently behind bars.[6] This has occurred despite an overall decrease in crime rates and has largely been the product of intensified harshness in sentencing and a focus on imprisonment over other forms of punishment. As David Cayley notes, "Incarceration rates are fed by the popular belief ... that punishment reduces crime, a belief seemingly immune to evidence."[7] Given the large body of evidence that this approach is a failure, it's an example of ideologically driven decision making trumping evidence-based policy. It also reflects a trend in Canada toward a less equal society, as Wilkinson and Pickett point out in *The Spirit Level:* "There is a strong social gradient in imprisonment, with people of lower class, income and education much more likely to be sent to prison than people higher up the social scale."[8] Corrections policies that emphasize incarceration reflect a worsening inequality and a growing tendency to view those of lower socio-economic status as dangerous, undeserving, and worthy of detention. The imprisonment of large numbers of marginalized people further marginalizes them, heightening the degree of social inequality.

Clearly, there is a problem here. The question is what to do about it. The big-picture answer is the theme of this book: work to create a healthy society, a more equal society, a fairer society, and you will have a safer society. This won't happen overnight, however, and it won't mediate the damage done by the current justice system. To alleviate the negative impact of the ill-named correction system, we need to significantly reform our approach to crime.

Safety in Numbers – The Evidence for Clemency

An effective justice system must measure its success mainly on how well it can change harmful behaviour into socially useful behaviour. We must reduce the techniques that have the side effect of increasing crime. These techniques (incarceration being the most obvious example) are expensive. Keeping someone in jail for one year can cost anywhere from $50,000 to more than $150,000, depending on the level of security, whether the institution is provincial or federal, and whether the convict is male or female.[9] With just under forty thousand prisoners in Canada on any given day, that's at least $2.0 billion per year. If we factor in parole and other non-inmate custody services, Canadians paid $3.9 billion in correctional costs during the 2008–09 fiscal year.[10] How many at-risk youth could be helped and kept from offending with even a portion of that sum? Money saved through reform could be used to fund organizations that help people with multiple disadvantages avoid further trouble with the law.

Canada needs a criminal justice system that works, one that efficiently and accurately identifies individuals who harm other citizens and uses the most effective techniques for reducing their chance of re-offending. Our present system does not focus on effective measures; instead, it concentrates on incarceration in an attempt to frighten potential offenders. That technique has been worse than useless.

To understand why, we need to examine the possibility that a person, after release, will commit another offence (recidivism). In 2002, researchers in New Brunswick analyzed 111 separate, peer-reviewed studies that, in turn, studied over 400,000 offenders.[11] The question was, once all variables were removed (such as sex, age, race), what is the difference between similar individuals who are sentenced to prison terms and those who are placed on probation and allowed to live at home? The clear answer was that the former were 3 to 7 percent more likely than the latter to reoffend after being released. The longer the jail time, the higher the chance of reoffending: among individuals who were incarcerated for more than two years, recidivism increased an average of 7 percent.

There are many reasons for sending people to prison, but we can't rely on detention to reduce future crime – that conclusion is inescapable. Incarceration does not decrease crime. It increases it and thus makes us less safe. This dangerous side effect helps explain why democratic, wealthy countries have differing rates of incarceration that correspond to differing crime rates. For example, the United States jails several times more people per capita than do Canada, Germany, and Japan.[12] Its per capita rate of murder and other serious crimes is also several times greater than that of Canada, Germany, and Japan.[13] My home province of Saskatchewan incarcerates more youth per capita than almost all other wealthy, democratic nations.[14] We are moving toward disaster.

The majority of Canadian spending on reducing future harms goes to incarceration. If there are more effective techniques for diminishing crime, doesn't it make sense to stop channelling our tax dollars into one that encourages it, when we could allocate the money saved to crime reduction techniques instead?

To further explore how the determinants of health shape involvement in the justice system, and exactly how just that system is, it is useful to ask who goes to jail. Incarcerated youth in Saskatchewan tend to be different from those who are never incarcerated. The most obvious difference is the number and seriousness of the problems they inherit. They are far behind their peers in school; by the age of twelve or thirteen, almost all are roughly one to three years behind students of the same age.[15] Functional illiteracy is common, as it is in adult jails. Eighty percent of them have a disability – some are less serious learning disabilities, whereas others are more profound such as ADHD and fetal alcohol spectrum disorders.[16] Ninety percent come from families that live in poverty.[17] Over 80 percent are of a minority race, the vast majority Indigenous.[18] More than half have had Social Services as their parent for at least some of their lives.[19] This latter statistic is particularly problematic. When parents run into trouble, rather than helping them keep their children, we take them away and put them in foster care. After the children are damaged by being separated from their families – and often by their experience of foster care – we don't help them stay out of trouble. We imprison them. This reactive response perpetuates the damage to families, particularly Métis and First Nations families harmed over generations through the reserve system, residential schools, and prolonged poverty, ensuring future generations of apprehended and incarcerated children. Former Assembly of First Nations national chief Shawn Atleo made headlines when he stated that children who grow up on reserves are more likely to go to prison than to finish high school,[20] a statistic that can only be seen as a stain on the nation's reputation. Clearly, something must be done to turn this situation around.

One promising crime prevention model is the Hub and Centre of Responsibility (COR) approach developed in Prince Albert, Saskatchewan, and now being emulated in more than two dozen Canadian cities.[21] This collaboration between police, corrections, social work, education, addictions, and mental health was inspired by similar efforts in Scotland that used a public health approach to reducing violent crime in Glasgow.[22] It sprang from the observation that people who were in trouble or at risk were often being seen by multiple sectors, which were neither communicating with each other nor co-ordinating their efforts. The Hub is a multi-sector meeting table designed to allow organizations to collaborate quickly in reaction to a crisis. A support unit for this work, the COR includes representatives from the various sectors, who use data and the best available evidence to track patterns and recommend system changes to improve community health and safety. When one of the agencies involved in the Hub identifies an individual or family that is at risk, it tries to help on its own. If it thinks that one of the other agencies could also help, it brings the information to the Hub table to ask for the advice and involvement of partners from other sectors.

Research, especially from health, education, and youth-oriented community groups, shows that more can be done, that we can work with these young people. Indeed, since groups such as Str8Up have as one of their goals encouraging youth to achieve their potential, they tend to transform these youth into successful citizens. Canada is fortunate to have many examples of effective programs, ranging from art education to conflict resolution, from employment education to canoeing with cops, from money management to drama. The more young people can

A Healthy Society

be shown the process that leads from disadvantage to success, and just how enjoyable it can be, the less likely they are to commit crimes. Unfortunately, most such organizations are starved for funds – living grant-to-mouth, as it were – so their impact is not as great as it might be. Given the high connection between substance abuse, crime, and mental and physical illness in Canada, taking a cue from Iceland and scaling up from small, successful projects to a robust, nationwide strategy for active young people would be a worthwhile investment in our future.[23]

An effective justice system must measure its success mainly on how well it changes harmful behaviour to social usefulness. To do that, we must invest in crime prevention and curtail punitive practices that have the unintended effect of increasing crime. The money saved should be used to fund organizations that can help youth with multiple disadvantages not only to survive but to thrive. It can also help prisons focus on rehabilitation. Building in intensive counselling and skills training, and creating privilege- and sentence-related incentives that promote success in rehabilitation can make prisons into actual corrections facilities that prepare inmates for a better, more responsible life on the outside rather than perpetuating criminal culture.

If we want a safer society, we need to aim for effective measures that really reduce crime and rely less on trying to frighten the marginalized. We need to use the available evidence to transform our justice system into a force for good. Again, we see the parallel with health care, where what we currently have are revolving-door clinics, treating people when they are ill and dealing with symptoms but failing to ask why they get sick in the first place. This guarantees that they'll be back and sick again, just as a justice system that treats the symptom of crime with the medication of prison and fails to address the root causes of criminal behaviour ensures that we will have revolving-door prisons. Some suggest that we should mete out longer and tougher sentences; however, as the evidence shows, this merely exacerbates the problem and increases repeat crime and incarceration. How much wiser would it be to work with people to get them out of the justice system than to keep them in as long as possible?

Coming back to Brad Peequaquat, I am struck by the enormous waste of opportunity. Here was a young man who tried to turn his life around. He sought help, but the system responded with negligence, blindly enforcing the rules. The result has been considerable financial cost for both the hospital and the justice system, the tragedy of pain, disability, and ultimately death for Brad, and great sadness for his family. For all of us, it means the loss of a bright young man, who, given the opportunity, could have helped others to see that there were better choices than street life.

The implications of the parallels between justice and health are profound. The same factors that make us sick – poverty, unemployment, poor education, substandard housing, and lack of nutrition – predict our likelihood of incarceration. It stands to reason that, if we invest in people's health and well-being, we will also be investing in crime prevention and the safety of all citizens. Saskatoon chief of police Clive Weighill suggested that "we need to get tough on poverty, poor housing, racism – the social issues that lead us down the road to crime."[24] Finding creative ways to do just this will keep people out of the justice system and keep our streets safe at the same time.

9

LEARNING TO LIVE

In the neighbourhood where I work, there are a lot of women who live in difficult circumstances. Some come regularly to the clinic, seeing it as a safe place where people want to help. Others choose different organizations such as EGadz Street Outreach, AIDS Saskatoon, or Quint Development Corporation. And some don't, can't, or won't seek help at all. Amy is one of the latter, a twenty-six-year-old mother of three who hasn't been doing well. She's on social assistance, in an abusive relationship, and addicted to alcohol. Whether it's the strength of her addiction, her controlling partner, or just a lack of belief that anyone will help her, she's been reluctant to get help. I see her occasionally in the clinic for acute issues, but she doesn't stay engaged or keep follow-up appointments, and she refuses offers of help to get out of her current situation. People like Amy can be frustrating because there are ways to help them, but they aren't ready to change, and there's little we can do to move them toward readiness.

There have been times when I've seen more of Amy and when she was a bit more willing to consider a new life. This wasn't because of anything we'd done at the clinic; it's due to her cousin, Mason. Mason works as an engineer, is politically and socially active, and is generally a pretty together young man. When you hear about how he grew up, the unlikeliness of this becomes obvious. Alcohol, drugs, poverty, and petty crime were around him all the time. His father died from the complications of a lifelong alcohol addiction. Many of his relatives are in prison or

131

imprisoned by poverty and addictions. The question that stories like Mason's always bring to mind is, why did he bounce when those around him fell flat? Why is he succeeding when so many of his cousins, peers, and friends have ended up in situations as bad or worse than that of the generation before them? He's a healthy young man enjoying a good life, but many of the determinants of health in his upbringing – income, social status, physical environment – worked against that. Why was he able to take the hardships and use them as reasons to succeed rather than excuses not to?

Mason attributes it to the fact that, when things got really bad with his parents, he went to stay with his maternal grandfather, a math and history teacher. Life at his grandfather's was different: there was enough to eat, they weren't constantly moving, and no one was drunk. In these more peaceful times, Mason's grandfather taught him how to learn and helped him develop a talent for math. Math became his escape when things got bad and eventually the balloon that lifted him up where no one thought he'd go.

Though school was a struggle for him socially – he was often excluded because of his race and status – he could count on getting decent marks. At university he found a more welcoming social scene and thrived in the college of engineering. Now he has a successful job as an engineer, and he works with young people in Saskatoon's inner city, tutoring math and helping others find the talent that will move them out of poverty and despair.

Mason is a remarkable individual, but according to him one thing is clear: school helped. He was fortunate enough to live in Saskatchewan, one of the few places in the world where the rich and the poor send their kids to public school, where there is no distinction between the good school and the bad school. There is just school. And Mason had talented teachers, including his grandfather, who recognized his potential and challenged him along the way. When he struggled, he got extra help; when he was bored, he was challenged.

Education is recognized as one of the key determinants of health. The higher the level of education someone can achieve, the more likely they are to live a longer and healthier life. Like income, it also has an impact on the other determinants. Level of education is strongly

A Healthy Society

correlated with income, as those with more training and skills can command higher levels of pay and better employment opportunities and working environments. The literacy and numeracy skills obtained through education influence how people access housing and health care, as well as their choices regarding nutrition, physical activity, smoking, and substance use. Social skills acquired during schooling aid the formation of social support networks.

The process of education, both curricular and informal, is in general one that contributes to a healthy life. Where there is a common public school system, accessible to everyone, education is a force for greater equality in society. Horace Mann notes, "Education then, beyond all other devices of human origin, is the great equalizer of the conditions of men, the balance-wheel of the social machinery."[1]

A Class Apart

The degree to which education is effective in its role as equalizer depends on the same elements as health care does: access, quality, and affordability. In most of Canada, we are still fortunate enough to have good public schools, but gaps in access and quality are cause for concern, especially where private or charter schools are more prevalent. There are inequities between rural and urban schools at all levels, as well as differences in quality of education and extra-curricular opportunities, depending on community incomes.

One example of a growing gap is the condition of schools on First Nations reserves. In the fall of 2011, the Cree nation of Attawapiskat declared a state of emergency that drew national attention, including a fundraising campaign through the Canadian Red Cross. Housing had deteriorated in quality and availability, with many of the 1,500 band members living in poorly built, overcrowded shelters. These lacked indoor plumbing and adequate insulation and heating to withstand a northern Ontario winter. The housing crisis was only the latest in a long list of troubles for Attawapiskat, including insufficient water treatment facilities and pollution from a large diesel spill under the elementary school. The spill caused health problems among children and teachers, and the school was demolished, as it should have been. What didn't follow was a new school. Successive federal governments refused to build a replacement, prompting community youth to start a campaign, which has become known as Shannen's Dream.[2] It is named after Shannen Koostachin, an Attawapiskat student champion who, prior to her death in a car accident at age fifteen, was nominated for the International Children's Peace Prize as a representative of the children who advocated for a new school.

Referring to the lack of a school at Attawapiskat, Charlie Angus, MP for Timmins-James Bay, Ontario, asked, "What other Canadian kid has to fight, organize and beg for access to clean and equitable schools?"[3] The story of Attawapiskat is a particularly strong example of the inequality of experience and opportunity faced by First Nations children. In a time of population growth among First Nations people, Indian and Northern Affairs Canada placed a 2 percent per year growth cap on education spending, effectively legislating long-term underfunding.[4] On average, on-reserve schools are funded a third less per student than schools elsewhere in Canada – all of this when Aboriginal students have the highest educational needs, including the lowest level of completion of secondary education, and schools in which students are described as being two grades behind those of comparable schools off-reserve.

This inattention and underfunding doesn't make a lot of sense. What teacher, presented with a student who was struggling, would deliberately give them a third less attention than the other students? In good classrooms, a student who is having difficulty receives more attention, and rightly so. Wise teachers know that the earlier they help a struggling student, the brighter the future for that student and the better the experience for the entire class. The same wisdom should be applied to addressing key determinants of health such as education among the communities most in need, be they urban, rural, or on-reserve; greater attention and resources should be applied to deal with greater challenges.

The Education Advantage

The challenges in education don't end at Grade 12. When young people enter the workforce, they face increased requirements for post-secondary education but greater impediments to their pursuit. Tuition fees have risen dramatically at universities across the country. Adding higher costs of living, particularly for students who must leave home to attend school, means youth from low-income families are simply unable to afford further training. For example, Saskatchewan has seen Western Canada's highest spike in tuition rates during the last decade.[5] At the same time, the number of students from low-income families enrolled in higher education has dropped precipitously.[6] Those who do attend carry debt burdens that hinder further study or becoming established in their careers and businesses. Student loan debt reduction has been falling, with provincial governments moving toward tax rebates for graduates. Although this appeals to governments, because it entails no increase in expenditures and can potentially entice graduates to stay in the province, it does nothing to reduce the up-front costs faced by students.

One striking change, which typifies the current direction but has gone largely without debate, is charging differential tuition for professional schools such as medicine and law. The idea that, since they will eventually earn more, students in these colleges should pay higher tuition (often two to three times that of students in other fields), makes sense on the surface. However, its ultimate effect is to exclude people from lower-income and non-urban families. Thus, education acts not as an equalizing force, but as something that preserves social difference. The result is not only less opportunity for those with greater needs, but also a less representative workforce in important fields of service. The medical school at the University of Manitoba has been trying to admit more people from economically disadvantaged backgrounds, setting aside spots for low-income students,[7] and the University of Saskatchewan plans to follow suit. However, this does not overcome the financial barrier to training, and heavy debt loads may push students to choose higher-paying specialties or practices. This tends to mean greater specialization and less work with marginalized populations, creating more barriers to equity in health service delivery.

An educated, healthy populace is our goal. It's also a positive feedback loop, an economic driver in itself. Removing barriers of access allows people to live fuller lives. It is also an investment in future prosperity, as healthy, educated people are better able to contribute to a society that produces healthy, educated people.

Canada has historically been a leader in public education investment, with affordable, quality institutions. However, during the budget crises of the 1990s, public investment was significantly cut and has never recovered to previous per capita levels.[8] This has affected access through rising tuition costs; it has also affected quality, with increased class sizes and reduced or eliminated key areas of study. Not only is this failure to invest in education unwise for the health of the population, it's also a strategic error economically. Tying ourselves to an economy that is based solely on natural resources is a backward step. Rather than being leaders in the emerging knowledge economy, we leave ourselves vulnerable to fluctuations in the commodity and labour markets. Investing in quality education will develop a generation with the skills not only to adapt to economic and technological advances but also to pioneer their development.

Learning to Learn

It is not enough to prepare learners for the workforce of today; we need to give them the skills to think critically and adapt to change in a world that may bear little resemblance to the one in which we currently live. Education is about more than simply obtaining the skills to succeed financially and live comfortably. Canadian educator and former Saskatchewan premier Woodrow Lloyd noted that education "is, or should be, concerned with changing the motivation that determines the direction of our seeking and moving so that society can be built on a firm foundation of human values ... Education should result not just in better trained hands and minds, but also in greater hearts."[9] There are facts to learn, of course, key concepts and information to digest and understand. More important, however, is learning literacy, the ability to apply critical thinking and skills in knowledge acquisition to adapt to a changing world. This requires literacy in household management, personal development, environmental stewardship, and in finding and creating employment.

It also applies directly to making personal health choices. An important element of making wise choices is health literacy, the ability to access, comprehend, and act on information for health. This ranges from simple things such as understanding immunizations or medications to making wise decisions in diet, exercise, and addictions, and being able to manage psychologically difficult periods of life, turning the anxiety and depression of tumultuous times into opportunities for personal growth.

People who have higher levels of education are more likely, on average, to land stable, well-paying jobs or to be successful in business. More and more jobs require higher levels of education. These facts cause confusion, as people conflate the results with the underlying purpose. They start to think that, because education leads to employment and material success, that's what it is for. As human beings, we are far more than our jobs and our bank accounts, and the goals of our learning must reflect a deeper sense of purpose. Perhaps the greatest goal of education is not a set of skills, but the development of values. Our democracy is only as healthy as the next generation of youth and its ability to engage creatively with the world. Civic literacy means teaching youth not to be future subjects, passive spectators of the news, but actors in the lives of their communities. The Saskatchewan Human Rights Commission has been taking the lead on this, developing a set of resources for teachers on citizenship education to be integrated into the provincial curriculum.[10]

One of the best ways for governments to perpetuate the ability to make bad decisions for the majority, with the support of the majority, is to diminish the quality of education. Some educational theorists, such as the University of Ottawa's Joel Westheimer, have suggested that this is one motivation for education reforms in the United States, and some parts of Canada, that emphasize standardized testing on defined facts and skills, reducing the time available for civic education and critical thinking.[11] School curricula in previous decades allowed space for the discussion of social and environmental concerns, often providing the fuel for student activism. This sort of content should be encouraged, as it can produce young people who are engaged with the world around them. It can inspire them to participate more fully in democracy and even to lead the kind of societal change that reflects the values taught in elementary school.

Currently, there is a disconnect between what we're taught in school and the values exhibited by people in positions of authority. It's a frequent observation that elected officials often behave in ways that no grade school teacher would accept. When my son Abraham came to watch me give my maiden speech in the legislature, he hid and refused to stay for Question Period because he was so angry with how rude everyone was to each other. Far worse than the childish behaviour of those who should be leaders are the narrow-minded and self-interested policy choices that would not pass the Grade 5 social studies smell test. No wonder that governments whose choices threaten our environment or oppress certain groups also tend to defund public education, undermining the ability of teachers to teach and students to learn.

To provide the kind of learning environment that will create more responsible future leaders, we need to value those who do the front-line work. As I wrote this chapter for the first edition, Saskatchewan's teachers had launched strike action for the first time in nearly eighty years. Typically, the media focused on wages and percentages; the teachers wanting more, the government offering less, and the public in the middle, wondering what was fair. As with most strikes, there were deeper questions that didn't make the headlines.

How do we value the work that teachers do? If we want our young people to have the best education, how do we make that happen? Obviously, we must attract bright, committed people to the teaching profession. This means not only valuing them by paying them well, but also by creating an environment in which they and their students can thrive. If teachers are to respond to and lead educational innovation, they must have opportunities to improve their skills and learn additional and emerging techniques throughout their careers. Rather than going backward to a more prescriptive and less responsive system of education, or playing hardball with teachers regarding their demands, we need to explore ways to advance the cause of learning at all levels.

Off to a Good Start

Early childhood experiences are key determinants of the health of children and the adults they will eventually become. The biggest impact on these experiences is material privation; the approximately 15 percent of Canadian children who live in poverty can expect an uphill climb when seeking healthy lives.[12] The interventions that have the greatest impact on childhood health will be economic: lifting families out of poverty. Paul Kershaw, economist at the University of British Columbia, describes the current generation that is raising children as "generation squeezed," as it faces increasing costs of living without an associated increase in wages. For example, housing costs across Canada grew by 76 percent between 1976 and 2006, whereas household incomes grew by only 6 percent, even though nearly twice as many women had joined the workforce during that period and were contributing to family incomes.[13]

The educational system has an important role to play, one that goes beyond custodial day care to providing quality experiences that help children develop the cognitive, language, and emotional skills to succeed in later life. In Saskatchewan, we are nowhere near meeting this goal. We have the lowest rate of child care availability in the country, with less than 10 percent of children under six being accommodated.[14] Aside from being inconvenient for single-parent families, or families in which both parents work, this child care deficit decreases opportunities for implementing structured early childhood learning, and it affects the provincial economy. In Quebec, the provincial government made child care available at $7.00 per day, a subsidy that increased the number of women in the workforce and contributed to tax revenue by $1.50 for each dollar invested.[15] This is another remarkable instance in which investment in human infrastructure pays for itself in the short term. It also has a long-term benefit to the children and their families, and ultimately to society as well, in terms of increased productivity and decreased social cost. Expanding the opportunities for early childhood education, from enhanced child care to all-day kindergarten, is a cost-effective and evidence-based means of improving public health.

One of the more interesting means of making these changes is the community school, or "School Plus" as it was called for a time in Saskatchewan. Community schools provide a focal point for neighbourhood services such as community associations, adult learning centres, pediatricians, nurses, psychologists, social workers, elders, addiction counsellors, and others. In the northern community of Île-à-la-Crosse, there is a particularly shining example of this model. A bright yellow building, designed to resemble a sunset, looks out over the lake toward the historic island for which the town is named. This unique facility is anchored by two main tenants: St. Joseph's Hospital and Rossignol High School. St. Joseph's is an acute care hospital with an emergency room, labs, an x-ray, and a long-term-care centre. Rossignol High School has classroom, lab, and physical education facilities for students from Grades 7 to 12. In addition to the hospital and the school, there are a family medicine clinic, mental health counsellors, public health offices, and a community-run child care and early learning centre. With a library and gymnasium, a performing arts stage, meeting rooms, and adult education classrooms, the Île-à-la-Crosse Integrated Services Centre is a one-stop-shop approach to addressing the determinants of health that expands the role of the school into a resource for everyone in the community, from newborns to elders.

Another appealing model is the integration of key services into existing facilities, as building new schools and hospitals is rarely an option. St. Mary's School in the inner-city Saskatoon neighbourhood of Pleasant Hill is host to a number of outreach initiatives from the local health region designed to address health inequities. These include an agility training program to address childhood obesity and inactivity, a nursing residency program that places nursing students in the classroom to work with children, and a pediatric clinic that offers clinical services in the school three days a week. Bringing the services to the children, rather than making families with limited means and multiple challenges come to appointments in other neighbourhoods, ensures that more kids get the help they need.

Higher Education

To free ourselves from the boom-and-bust cycle of our resource-based economies, we need to ready ourselves for the knowledge economy of the future. Investment in K-12 education must be coupled with investment in post-secondary education, including professional colleges and technical schools, as well as basic sciences and humanities. Post-secondary education is one of the investments with the greatest return for governments. For example, the University of Saskatchewan has a fiscal multiplier of 1.35 for the Saskatchewan economy, which is to say that for every dollar spent on post-secondary education, $1.35 is returned to the provincial economy, approximately $1,000 per Saskatchewan resident in total.[16] Of course, this constitutes only the immediate return to the economy. It doesn't account for the long-term value to our economic and physical health of having young people who have been able to pursue the knowledge and skills that higher education provides.

Poverty has always been a barrier to post-secondary education. With increasing tuition and related fees, a lack of affordable housing, and the rising cost of nutritious food, post-secondary education is a challenge for young people from middle-class and working families.[17] Many choose not to pursue it. Those who do often graduate with a burden of debt that will take most of their working lives to pay off.

Education must be affordable and accessible for every young Canadian. While tax credits may be a valuable means of keeping graduates in regions where they are needed, they are of little use if the cost of education keeps people out of school in the first place.[18] Lowering barriers to post-secondary training, like subsidizing early childhood education, is an investment that pays off quickly in productivity and tax revenue, and should be a priority for provincial and federal governments. This can be done by reducing tuition rates, increasing the number and amount of scholarships, targeting under-represented populations, simplifying and forgiving more student loans, and providing support to students who must move to larger centres to continue their education. Taking affordable, practical steps to make education more accessible will allow us to prepare coming generations to lead us in advancing the health and well-being of all people.

In the first edition of the book, I ended this chapter with an update on Amy. At the time, she'd moved into a new apartment and hadn't had a drink for over a month. Her partner was enrolled in anger management classes, and she was thinking about going back to school. Although this change was her own success, she did attribute some of it to her cousin Mason's influence. By taking her kids for breaks, connecting Amy to the clinic, and just staying present in her life, he showed her a different way to live. The success of one family member through education was a bridge to a better life, evidence that there are smarter and healthier ways to live.

Unfortunately, in this second edition I have to add a less happy postscript to that ending. After a few years of practice, I noticed that a certain pattern repeated itself among some of my most challenging patients. They would get things together and manage to live in healthier ways, start to show promise of a happier life, but then something would go wrong: a family member would get sick, they'd meet up with a partner who wasn't good for them, their housing would change, or they'd simply slip up and start using again. This is incredibly hard to watch, as we invest our hope in people's recoveries. We want them to get better and stay that way, and it's heartbreaking to see things spiral. Over time, I found that the best way of dealing with this was to think of it differently. When people start from the bottom, falling down is not failure – getting up is success. When they have windows of clarity, of reconnection with family, of even the dream of a job or a stable home, that's what we need to celebrate, even after things have gone badly. This is analogous to the human condition: all of us represent brief windows of life that, when finished, are better celebrated than mourned.

Amy's window lasted a little while, but then her relationship with her partner and with substances got the better of her again. I saw her the other day on the street, skinny and sick and lost. She's alienated from most of her family, including Mason. There is always hope for another window, for a revival and a reconnection, but the reality is that our early lives stay with us forever. The combination of childhood traumatic events – of which she experienced many – and the loss of opportunity from not being able to continue with school made her permanently vulnerable. It's a tragic reminder that the more we do to keep kids safe and in school, the greater their ability to rebound from tough times. Investing collectively in learning, from early childhood to ongoing training, makes us all smarter and healthier.

10

HEADING DOWNSTREAM

> By addressing the social determinants of health you can
> provide better care and save money.
>
> — Jeff Turnbull, "Building a Stronger, Sustainable
> Medicare for Canadians"[1]

Early in my medical career, I spent a few years working as what is called
a *locum tenens*, which is Latin for place-holder. Essentially, I was a book-
mark in the practice stories of other physicians, giving them a break
and making sure that the people they worked for could still see a doctor.
This was an exciting job. It introduced me to new towns, new people,
and new ways of practising medicine. With a fascinating mix of emergency, clinic, and long-term care, in facilities new to me, it also kept me
on my toes.

Of the many challenging situations, there is one that particularly
sticks out. The day after Boxing Day in 2008, I was staying in a small
town west of Saskatoon. At around ten thirty in the evening, a lady named
Lynn Peters, who was experiencing chest pain and difficulty breathing,
came into the emergency room. She'd had the same thing before and
had wound up in hospital but wasn't sure what the cause had been.

Her legs were swollen. I listened to her lungs. They sounded a little
bit wet, probably mild pulmonary edema. Those two together often

mean heart failure. An ECG, an electrical tracing of her heart, showed the classic "tombstone" shape that indicates a myocardial infarction: a heart attack. I talked to the cardiologist on call in Saskatoon and faxed her the ECG to double-check. She agreed it looked like a heart attack, and we decided, given the distance to Saskatoon, to try TNK, a clot-busting medication. Heart attacks are caused by blood clots in the arteries that feed the heart. When they're plugged, the heart muscle starts to die. TNK breaks down the clot to open up blood flow to the heart. Done in time, this essentially reverses the heart attack and helps prevent serious damage. I'd never used it before, so the cardiologist reviewed the steps with me, and then I did what happens so often in the field. I tried something I'd only read about.

This time, it failed. Whether as a result of or despite the TNK, Lynn's breathing suddenly got worse. Far worse. Her lungs now sounded as if they were underwater, and pink foam was coming from her mouth. Her blood oxygen levels had dropped from 98 percent to 60 percent, even though she was wearing an oxygen mask at full flow. I would have to put in a tube to help her breathe.

This I'd done before, but not since residency, not in this hospital, and never without a more experienced doctor present. Once again, I chose to phone a friend. Despite the late hour, I called one of my classmates, an emergency physician who does intubations all the time. I told him my plan. He gave me some tips on how much of which medicine would paralyze Lynn's muscles and make her unconscious while the nurses adjusted her position and got the equipment ready. Whether due to my inexperience or because her tongue and throat were extremely swollen, I couldn't get her tubed, not even with special instruments, and neither could the ambulance staff. At one point, her oxygen levels dropped into the forties, and I found myself running around the unfamiliar emergency room, looking for a scalpel in case I had to cut into her trachea and create an emergency airway.

Fortunately, I managed to insert a laryngeal mask airway (a rescue breathing device that works nearly as well as the tube I was trying to use) and get her oxygen saturation back up to 90 percent with a bag-valve mask, squeezing each breath into her lungs. We kept squeezing the bag while we moved her into the back of the ambulance and set off for Saskatoon, speeding down the potholed highway in minus 35 degree weather. During the two- and a half-hour trip, we took turns breathing for her. Miraculously, we managed to keep the mask in place, despite the bumps, and Lynn stayed clinically stable all the way to the Royal University Hospital, where the emergency team took over, the anesthesiologist intubated her, and the cardiologists went to work to see what could be done for her heart and lungs.

A couple of days later, I finished my service in that town and came back to Saskatoon, so I went to the hospital to see how Lynn was doing. When I walked into her room, she was sitting up in bed, having lunch. Her breathing was fine. I had to introduce myself because she didn't remember anything of what had happened that night. All she knew was that she came into hospital feeling sick, and now she was in Saskatoon feeling good, anxious to be discharged home.

This is an example of the most exciting and thrilling part of health care: using the skills of the health care team and the resources of the system to save people from the brink of death. Even for the trained and practised, it's scary as hell. In many ways, avoiding emergencies and all the times when people aren't as lucky as Lynn is the point of this book. Her story, however, illustrates the importance of downstream care as one element of ensuring a healthy population.

As I mentioned earlier, health services are far down the list of the determinants of health, and much of this book is about making political changes to avoid health problems. It is estimated that non-health-care determinants account for three-quarters or more of health outcomes.[2] However, the other quarter is important, and downstream responses still have a significant role in addressing quality of life. They're a safety net that comes into play when prevention and primary care fail, and can also teach us much about that failure. The number of people who access emergency rooms, are diagnosed with major illnesses, or need surgery is an accurate indicator of how well our upstream work is succeeding.

Of course, this measurement must be taken carefully. Like GDP growth, general improvements in health outcomes can be misleading, masking deep inequalities. The overall trend in Canada is toward greater longevity, but in many parts of the country those at the bottom of the socio-economic scale are sicker and dying sooner. Public health research needs to be thorough and creative to use illness statistics to draw a clear picture of Canadian health.

One way of ensuring that the right treatment is available for those who are ill is to have a health care system that is, as described in the Canada Health Act, universal, comprehensive, accessible, portable, and publicly administered. Designing services, from immunization programs to surgical wards, that meet the priority health concerns of those most in need can contribute significantly to improvements in health status.

To begin, we must recognize a couple of things about the current system. First, great strides have been made. The introduction of Medicare, a universal program for all Canadians, is one of the most remarkable accomplishments of our nation. It has resulted in better and fairer provision of health services, as well as a better understanding of the health problems faced throughout the country. Second, we must also acknowledge that the system is not perfect. Access and delivery can be inefficient, and barriers to change make it costlier and less effective than it could be.

Care Where and When It's Needed

When we were expecting our first child, my wife, Mahli, was doing an elective in adolescent medicine in Toronto as part of her pediatrics residency. She was five months pregnant and feeling unwell enough that she needed to see a doctor. We were reluctant to go to the hospital in a strange city, but we wanted to be sure that everything was all right. We went to the famous Mount Sinai hospital, walked into emergency, and were sent straight up to the obstetrics floor. We were well treated, all the appropriate tests were done, and in two hours we were heading home, reassured. At no time were we told that we weren't welcome because we came from another province, asked about our ability to pay, or made to feel that we were wasting time and money. We were amazed at the quality of care and ease of access.

In stark contrast is an experience from a few years ago. I was visiting friends on a First Nations reserve in northern Saskatchewan. It was mid-February and about minus 20, and I decided to go cross-country skiing on the frozen lake. After about half an hour, a man drove up on a snowmobile.

"Are you the doctor?" he asked.

I said yes, assuming he recognized me from previous visits and just wanted to say hi.

"Get on, there's been an accident."

We sped into town to the clinic, which is staffed by two very capable registered nurses and has a weekly "doctor day," when a doc from a nearby town flies in to see the patients whom the nurses are concerned about. There we found Brandon, a teenager who'd been in a traffic accident. He'd been the passenger on a quad – a four-wheel all-terrain vehicle – that had slid into the back of a truck at the only stop sign in town. He was thrown into the path of an oncoming truck and run over. Barely conscious, he had two broken legs and a pretty serious head injury. I worked with the nurses and a medical student who was also visiting the reserve to prepare him for transport. As a team, we splinted his legs, stabilized his neck, started lines, and got him into an ambulance, which sped down the gravel road to a town an hour away. From there, he was flown another hour to Saskatoon for surgery and weeks of rehabilitation. As a team, we'd turned Brandon's very bad luck slightly better, making a potentially fatal accident into something he'd recover from in time.

Like most doctors, I have a collection of this kind of story, of being in the right place at the right time. But I'm painfully aware of how often the opposite must be true. It was pure chance that we were there visiting and could help Brandon. There are stories from across the country, in small towns, inner-city neighbourhoods, and on reserves, where people aren't as lucky, where access to health care is neither timely nor reliable. The recruitment of trained professionals is difficult in more remote communities, and many who are recruited come for brief periods, don't understand local issues, and may actually impede the delivery of quality care. If health services are to function properly, they must be delivered when and where they're needed. Unfortunately, that is not the case for the poorest third of Canadians.[3]

Responding to the Needs of Society

Fully aware of these issues, Saskatchewan's medical school has been host to the Division of Social Accountability for the past several years. Social accountability, as defined by the World Health Organization, is the obligation of medical schools to "meet the priority health needs of the communities they serve."[4] The division attempts to identify unmet health needs in Saskatchewan and beyond, and to direct the activities of the medical school in clinical activity, advocacy, research, and education and training (known as the CARE model) to address them.[5] This work has resulted in, among other things, the creation of some innovative programs to teach medical students about service.

One program that exposes students to real life situations with the intention of giving them a deeper understanding of the determinants of health is called Making the Links. Students in this program volunteer at SWITCH, the student-run clinic in inner-city Saskatoon. They also work in northern Saskatchewan communities, including the reserve where Brandon was injured. In the final phase of the program, they work in Mozambique, Uganda, or Vietnam. Through these varied experiences, with rural and remote Aboriginal communities, in an underserved urban setting, and in a lower-resource country, the students become intimately familiar with the ways in which social determinants affect people's health. By participating in this community service learning, contributing to the local communities while learning about the health issues they face, students move beyond hearing about dry concepts in a classroom setting to making real connections with people and their stories. These personal and meaningful relationships create a deeper understanding of patients as people and of the factors in their lives that determine whether or not they'll be healthy.

Although this program has a huge impact on individual students, its scope is small. If we really want health care services to be offered where and how they're needed, substantial changes will be required. Some will occur in training, with more physicians, nurses, and other professionals being trained in the communities that most need service. This will produce greater understanding of rural or inner-city life and will develop relationships with and affinity for communities, ultimately prompting more people to serve where they are needed.

The way in which health care is provided and paid for also needs to change. Typically, physicians are paid "fee-for-service," with each patient visit being charged to the government. This results in some perverse incentives away from the best quality care. For example, in Saskatchewan a clinic visit is classified as a 5B, and it pays the same amount whether it deals with a cold or a new diagnosis of cancer. As you can imagine, these visits take very different amounts of time, knowledge, and concentration. In essence, the system encourages speedy care of minor problems and the avoidance of complexity. Shifting to salary or mixed payment schedules encourages physicians to spend more time at the front end of care, assessing all the issues of a patient before they get out of hand. This would also correct the major discrepancy between the pay of specialists and that of the family doctors on the front line.

Reform in the way that physicians, nurses, pharmacists, physiotherapists, and others work together can also make a big difference. By pooling their efforts, primary health care teams can offer a holistic approach to patient care. This means more co-ordinated care, wiser use of the skills of highly trained professionals, and more attention to patient experience and what's really needed to make a difference.

As Sustainable as We Want It to Be

As a result of public administration, the cost of doctor and hospital services is relatively stable. Each has fallen as a portion of the total spending on health (private and public) in the country. So why are health costs taking up ever-larger portions of provincial budgets?

The idea that other priorities are being displaced by ballooning health care costs is worth direct attention. We've recognized the importance of the determinants of health, of education, housing, and so on. If paying for health care consumes so much of our budget that spending on other priorities becomes impossible, that's unacceptable. Fortunately, we are not in this situation. Although some fluctuations have occurred, health care spending as a percentage of GDP has remained stable across the country since the 1970s.[6] The problem is not so much that spending has risen – it's that revenues have fallen. Through successive tax cuts and decreased royalty rates, the budgets of provincial governments have diminished. When you decrease revenue but don't change spending, the percentage goes up – it's not that health is taking a larger portion of the pie; the pie has shrunk. The portion covered by the federal government has also decreased, meaning that the health budget numbers show up at the provincial level instead. The truth remains, as former Saskatchewan premier Roy Romanow stated in the 2002 report of the Commission on the Future of Health Care in Canada, that "the system is as sustainable as we want it to be."[7] The question is whether the political will exists to change the direction of shrinking public revenue and investment and to reestablish the appropriate balance between provincial and federal contributions.

This threat of unsustainability is the constant, and most compelling, cry of those who would establish a private health care system in parallel to Medicare. Driven by the belief that health care is a commodity that can best be delivered by for-profit ventures, they argue that the current system would be aided – not endangered – by this change. The evidence is clear: this is rubbish. Wherever it has been tried (in other countries and in limited ways here in Canada), a parallel system has increased waiting lists and practitioner shortages in the public system. It also erodes commitment to funding the public system by those who can afford to sidestep the queues, ultimately engendering two systems that are very different in quality and cost. This debate, and the evidence that argues against moving toward privatization, is worth an entire book in itself – and there are many works to that effect, such as the Romanow Report and *Profit Is Not the Cure*, a popular work by Maude Barlow.[8]

However, even when we stand up for Medicare, we need to be careful. Too often, the threat of privatization evokes defensiveness among those who know the superiority of a single-payer, publicly funded system. We find ourselves entrenched in our positions and sticking up for the status quo. To build a healthy society, and to move out of this deadlock, we must stop defending Medicare. We must work to expand and improve our universal coverage.

One of the first steps is to realize just how little of our health care actually is public. Commentators on Medicare often compare Canada to North Korea and Cuba, citing them as the only other countries in which private health care does not exist. Though this is a provocative point, it's also a joke. In our system, only hospital and physician services are really publicly funded. Everything else is a mix of private and public, with the lion's share being private. In fact, when compared with other OECD countries, Canada actually has a far lower proportion of public funding in key areas. For example, though over 90 percent of physician and hospital services are publicly funded, that's true of only 39 percent of pharmaceuticals and 5 percent of dental services. By way of comparison, the German government funds 74 percent of drug costs and 61 percent of dental care. Our overall public spending on health care, at about 70 percent, is near the bottom of the pack of OECD countries.[9]

The costs of doctors and hospitals, the elements of the supposedly unsustainable public health care system, have actually remained fairly stable in absolute dollars. This means that, as a percentage of total health care expenditures, they have decreased considerably. The real cost drivers are those segments that lie almost entirely outside the public system. The largest culprit in this regard has been prescription drugs, the fastest-growing cost in health care budgets, both personal and public. In 2009, Canadians spent $30 billion on pharmaceuticals.[10] Many patients have told me that the price of multiple medications they need to manage illnesses such as diabetes is simply beyond their means. There is a pressing need for a strategy to decrease costs for the system and improve access for individuals.

In the past, even as recently as 2012, when this book was first published, national pharmacare was seen as too great a cost during a time of low political appetite for new universal benefits. But new research has revealed that pharmacare isn't a money sucker – it's a money saver. A closer look at the numbers shows that the cost of not having national drug coverage is far greater than that of implementing it. A groundbreaking economic analysis conducted in the spring of 2015 by Steve Morgan and his colleagues demonstrated that universal drug coverage would save over $7 billion in private and public spending, with little or no increase to government budgets.[11]

Where do these savings come from? Canada is the only OECD country whose universal health care program doesn't include drug coverage, which means that we don't get value for money when we buy medicine. The popular anti-cholesterol drug Lipitor, for example, costs nearly ten times as much for a Canadian patient as it does in New Zealand, where bulk buying and aggressive price negotiations are part of a national drug plan.[12] This means that Canadians are either paying far more out-of-pocket for drugs, or they're simply not buying them at all.

In my practice, as in medical practices across the country, I see patients with chronic illnesses such as diabetes, high blood pressure, HIV, and lung disease who are too often forced to choose between the medications that will keep them well and the necessities of life, such as rent and food. This problem in not unique to very low-income Canadians – it spans income lines, as drugs become more expensive and employer benefits less common. Doctors are so concerned about the issue that in 2015 the Canadian Medical Association's General Council voted 92 percent in favour of a resolution in support of pharmacare.

The general public agrees: recent polls show that 91 percent of Canadians support universal drug coverage.[13] We should not be surprised by this sentiment: according to an Angus Reid poll, in nearly a quarter of surveyed Canadian households, someone had skipped doses, cut pills in half, or simply not filled a prescription because the cost of medication was so high.[14] Obviously, this is bad for the immediate health of these individuals, but it also contributes to greater costs in other parts of the health system when patients suffer preventable consequences.

Getting in on the Action

The need for universal drug coverage is widely recognized and has re-newed calls to attenuate the runaway costs in this least-controlled segment of the health system. How prescriptions are to be paid for has been much debated. Should it be individually, through out-of-pocket expenses and insurance plans, or collectively, through taxation? Should all medications be covered, or should coverage be restricted to catastrophic events or specific age groups? The calls and evidence for universal pharmacare, guided by an evidence-based formulary, are growing ever stronger.

A related issue to covering and controlling the cost of drugs is the question of who makes them. Many are available in generic forms, produced at a fraction of the cost of the original manufacturer's product. Generic companies then sell the medications at a small discount off the price of brand-name product, which is to say that the profit margin on generic drugs is very high.

Leaving aside for a moment the question of who will pay for medications, what if they were made by governments?

Like many provinces in Canada, my home province of Saskatchewan has a long history of successful Crown corporations. They effectively and profitably provide essential services, such as vehicle insurance, telephone services, and electricity, and they sport patriotic names such as SaskTel and SaskPower.

Let's consider for a moment a hypothetical Crown corporation that produces generic drugs: SaskPharm. By establishing SaskPharm, Saskatchewan could supply essential medicines to its population, create local jobs, and save provincial health dollars. SaskPharm could manufacture and provide generic prescription drugs to Saskatchewan Health at cost, greatly decreasing procurement expenses. These savings could be applied to other parts of the health care system or invested in research and development. SaskPharm products could also be prescribed by doctors and sold to the public at a moderate profit. This would pass savings on to consumers while still furnishing operating and expansion capital. In addition, medications could be sold at bulk prices to other provinces and jurisdictions, along the lines of existing arrangements between provincial governments and generic pharmaceutical companies. This would result in savings to other provincial governments while creating further revenue streams for SaskPharm.

The potential economic benefits of such an approach are many. SaskPharm would generate jobs in research, medicine, information technology, commerce, and numerous other spin-off sectors, such as new markets for agricultural crops that can be transformed into medication. The development of this economic niche could provide jobs for Saskatchewan's young, growing population and attract professionals and business people from elsewhere.

If SaskPharm proved profitable in producing and selling generic drugs, it could potentially begin to research and develop new ones. This is perhaps the most exciting aspect of this idea. Other pharmaceutical companies profit only by selling their products: if people stop getting sick, they stop making money. As an arm of the provincial government, SaskPharm would profit by making or keeping people healthy. There would be a built-in incentive to tailor drugs specifically for the health conditions of the Saskatchewan people, such as new ways of monitoring or treating diabetes or helping to control the province's growing HIV epidemic. This would free up provincial funds for other priorities and would create potential for substantial profit from sales of SaskPharm original medications to other jurisdictions.

As it did with the introduction of universal health insurance, Saskatchewan could once again take a leadership role by forming a Crown corporation to develop and produce new medications. Saskatchewan is an ideal place to conduct this experiment: its market is large enough to warrant the investment, yet small enough that change would not be exceedingly cumbersome.

Clearly, this sort of innovation is not without its challenges. The start-up costs for market studies, establishing business plans, and obtaining accurate scientific information, methods of production, and personnel would require a major financial commitment, as would building a production site. Eventually, however, this expenditure could be offset by provincial savings in medication costs and the modest profit on sales to consumers.

The challenges are daunting, to say the least. Extreme care would need to be taken in relation to patent laws and trade agreements to ensure that no legal backlash arose. Competition would be fierce, and we could expect bitter marketing and legal battles, though this would be attenuated somewhat by the fact that Saskatchewan has no drug-production companies. But these risks are no greater than those faced by our predecessors when introducing Medicare, which began in one province and eventually expanded to the entire country. This is a different time, to be sure, but the appetite for inventive, evidence-based solutions in public policy remains strong. SaskPharm is a homegrown way of controlling drug costs in Saskatchewan and an approach that could be complementary to national pharmacare. It bears exploring. And perhaps CanPharm, and better health for all Canadians at lower cost, will be the eventual result.

Toward a Better Medicare

SaskPharm is just one provocative idea of how we can make the health care system more effective while containing costs. Others, such as creative wait times initiatives, expansion of home care, wider dental and vision care coverage, and long-term-care reform, are important ways of innovating in the system. Small-scale efforts across the country have shown how changes to the current system can improve the quality, accessibility, and affordability of care. We need to scale up those localized success stories to the national level, leading to a system that better responds to the needs of Canadians without compromising the integrity of the egalitarian enterprise of universal health insurance.

One hopeful driver of system change was the Health Council of Canada, a national body established at the time of the 2004–14 Canada Health Accord. The council's mission was to collect information about the performance of our health care system and to provide provincial and federal governments with guidance to improve surgical wait times, drug coverage during catastrophes, home care, primary health care, and electronic medical records. In its final major report – "Better Health, Better Care, Better Value for All" – the council described the years of the Health Accord as a decade in which the health system was failing Canadians.[15] This is strong language, and the council was emboldened by the Harper government's decision to close it down and to discontinue the accord. Still, in light of overall health spending in Canada, it's hard to argue with its view: private and public spending increased from $124 billion in 2003 to $228 billion in 2016 – no small sum.[16] But this new money brought little in the way of meaningful change in system performance or health outcomes for Canadians.

The blame for that doesn't rest with the council; it was consistent in its efforts to measure progress and point to new directions. No, the blame rests squarely on the shoulders of the provincial and federal leaders who authored the Health Accord. They failed to tie any of the increase in health funding to the innovations required to meet the stated goals. Rather than working together to scale up successes and learn from failures, the provinces set their own courses, with wide variation in degree of investment in innovation.

The Harper government then made a bad situation worse by walking away from the process of rebuilding a national health system instead of negotiating a more robust agreement with targets and timelines for innovation and cost savings.

The demise of the Health Council merely underlines this movement away from national planning for better outcomes. Were this a one-off elimination of a government body created for a short-term purpose, the decision would simply be disappointing. That the council's disappearance is part and parcel of a larger strategy to muzzle dissenting and unbiased voices – which are so necessary in a democracy – is downright disturbing.

By removing or limiting evidence-gathering bodies, be they in health, the environment, or general data such as the long-form census, we decrease the information available to us to shape our debate and decisions. By strictly controlling how scientists can share information, cutting public broadcasting, and terminating watchdog organizations such as the Health Council, we groom an ill-informed electorate. These backward steps are the recipe for bad decisions to be called good, for a poor-performing health care system, a weakened economy, and worsened health outcomes and quality of life for Canadians.

Canadians are proud of their health system and want to see it live up to its promise. Sooner or later, if governments are serious about delivering quality, accessible care, they'll have to come together to negotiate and co-operate. And they'll need an independent body to provide evidence and guidance on the best ways to do that. A great deal of work went into making the Health Council of Canada effective in its role; what a shame to have to start over from scratch.

My reason for highlighting various potential issues in the health care system, and the initiatives available to improve them, is to point out that the system is sustainable if we want it to be. And we should want it to be. In Chapter 4, I discussed the necessity of some degree of redistribution in the face of dangerous growth in inequality. Medicare is an active and effective form of redistributing wealth. Those who have benefitted most from our nation's wealth, and who in general have the good health to show for it, contribute to improving the health of those who have not. This is why Medicare is such a cornerstone of public policy in Canada and a perennially popular one among the general public. It's also why it encountered such virulent resistance upon introduction and continues to be under persistent, recurrent attack despite the overwhelming proof of its success.

These pressures and attacks will simply intensify as income equality grows. The poor and disadvantaged use a disproportionately higher amount of hospitals, medications, and physician services. In Saskatoon, residents of the low-income neighbourhoods use 35 percent more health care resources than the city's middle- and high-income residents, amounting to $179 million more per year in costs.[17]

This overall trend is set in even starker relief when we look at some of the individuals who require a great deal of medical support. The term "super utilizers," or "super users," was coined by Dr. Jeff Brenner of Camden, New Jersey, to describe people who, despite high levels of health intervention and expense, are still very sick.[18] His work also showed the existence of "medical hot spots" – specific areas in a community that often incur the highest health bills.

A 2014 report showed that just twenty individuals in Saskatoon were costing a total of $2 million per year in health and social services.[19] With a fifth of Saskatchewan's health expenditures going to serve just 1 percent of patients, it's no wonder that governments want to explore a different approach. Surely, there must be a more effective and less expensive way of helping those who are most in need.

Some of the answers may come from innovative models developed elsewhere. Jeff Brenner and others have used regular interdisciplinary team huddles, community-engaged outreach workers, and other creative means of adjusting the rigid world of health care delivery to meet the complex and chaotic needs of patients. These successes can teach us a great deal, but before we import too much from afar, we can look to some success stories of our own, including from my neighbourhood on the west side of Saskatoon. During an interview with CBC Radio's *White Coat Black Art* that described this part of the city as a medical hot spot, Jeff Brenner referred to two local initiatives mentioned earlier in this book – Station 20 West and SWITCH – as "disruptive change," the sort of delivery system game-changers required to address persistent, complex problems.[20] Other Saskatchewan successes include the Prince Albert Hub and COR model meetings that bring various agencies around a single table to help address the needs of high-risk families, as well as the multiple levels of housing and social support offered by Saskatoon's Lighthouse. The key to success in cooling medical hot spots lies in scaling up local interventions like these – and others across Canada – magnifying their strengths to help cope with the growing challenges of high-needs individuals.

Of course, addressing the needs of super users is only a first step. In many ways, these are the people we have already failed. Meeting their needs is essential, but we should also be trying to help prevent those who are currently struggling from becoming the super users of the future. Smart investments in the social determinants of health, including community economic development, can turn struggling neighbourhoods from medical hot spots into thriving, healthy communities.

This is a further reminder that, though health care is one way of redistributing wealth, it is not the most effective, coming as it does after people are already suffering the consequences of inequality. Failing to act sooner raises moral questions, such as why we are willing to help people when they're sick and dying but won't mobilize the resources to keep them healthy. It also poses a risk to the political feasibility of Medicare. When we don't address poverty and inequality, we create higher stress on our health care system. When we don't cover pharmaceutical costs or dental services, we increase expenses not only for individuals, but for the system as well. As people are unable to pay up front, or if primary health services aren't available and accessible, they get sicker and finally seek help later in the course of their illness. Just imagine the cost difference if we were to prevent diabetes or identify and treat it early rather than paying for the long hospital stays and kidney dialysis that are commonly required after the disease has progressed unchecked.

A system as fair and compassionate as Medicare needs to reflect a society that is also compassionate and fair. If all the weight of dealing with growing social inequality falls on the health care system, the cries of crisis will rise, and the commitment of those who are being asked to contribute more than they gain will continue to erode. Before long, we will find ourselves in a situation where patients like Lynn Peters or Brandon will be asked first, not "How can I help?" but "How will you pay?"

Much can be done to improve Medicare, but it must be accompanied by a concerted attempt to relieve pressure on the health care system by focusing on the rest of the determinants of health: income, education, physical environments, and more. This is how we can decrease costs in health care, improve access, and create the space needed to enhance quality. Only by working to keep people healthy can we hope to have a sustainable means of treating them when they are sick.

11

LESS POLITICS, MORE DEMOCRACY

It is only through such a system of global governance, placing fairness in health at the heart of the development agenda and genuine equality of influence at the heart of its decision-making, that coherent attention to global health equity is possible.

– Commission on Social Determinants of Health,
Closing the Gap in a Generation[1]

Change will demand the attention of all individuals, NGOs, business, communities, all levels of government and all sectors of our Canadian society. Success will require leadership from our prime minister and first ministers, from our mayors, municipal leaders, community leaders, and the leaders of our Aboriginal peoples. A whole-of-government approach is required with intersectoral action embracing business, volunteers, and community organizations. This will not be easy, but it can and must be done. We cannot afford to do otherwise.

– Senate of Canada, *A Healthy, Productive Canada*[2]

Slow Walk to Democracy

Several years ago, I accompanied a group of medical students from the University of Saskatchewan to Mozambique. We spent most of our time on the wards of the Massinga rural hospital, taking care of patients with malaria, HIV, pneumonia, and other serious conditions. Perhaps our most memorable experience, however, occurred far outside the walls of the hospital in the rural community of Tevele. For three days, we stayed in the homes of members of the Tevele health núcleo and took part in a survey of mosquito bed-net use.

Each morning, the students joined their group for a breakfast of bread and tea brought from town, and tangerines fresh from the tree. Then they walked from home to home. The groups, consisting of one or two Canadian students, two trainer students from the Centre for Continuing Education in Health, and several members of the núcleo, walked for many kilometres. They crossed rivers spanned by logs, trekked over hills and through brush, visiting all the families of the Tevele area. The families generally live in compounds of several small buildings with thatched roofs and walls of reeds or woven coconut palm leaves. At each house, the survey group would ask about who lived there, what methods they used to prevent malaria, and whether anyone had been sick with it in the past year.

This survey was part of a research relationship developed between the local people and the Training for Health Renewal Program (THRP), a partnership between the Canadian International Development Agency and the Mozambican Ministry of Health. THRP worked with Tevele for several years to establish the núcleo and thus to improve the overall health of the people in the area. Early on, representatives chosen by the various *círculos* that make up the Tevele area met with THRP and identified malaria as their number-one health priority. They then worked together to map the community and to perform an initial survey on malaria incidence and prevention methods. They discovered that very few people were using bed-nets to prevent mosquitoes from biting them and transmitting malaria.

The next step was to purchase and sell low-priced bed-nets to local people. The follow-up study showed that this had been quite successful at diminishing malaria. Many more families now faithfully protected themselves by sleeping under the nets, with pregnant women and young children appropriately getting priority use of them. When we conducted the follow-up survey, we asked those who had bed-nets where they had obtained them. Some mentioned Massinga or another town, but many said "Canada." This confused us until we discovered that it referred to the area under the big mango tree where the núcleo and THRP held their meetings. Community involvement at every step had resulted in the adoption of and pride in the project, a response that changed behaviour and saved lives by preventing malaria.

This kind of community development work is sometimes referred to as participatory action research.[3] Its key features are inherent in the name. It involves research, serious inquiry into the causes of ill health and the means to address them. The community participates fully in designing, directing, performing, and analyzing that research. Perhaps most importantly, the information that the project generates does not merely gather dust on a library shelf; it is translated into action that results in meaningful change for the community. The research, planning, action, and reflection in participatory action research are laborious and complicated. Much revision, reconsideration, and patience is required on the part of the núcleo members and the centre staff. The end result is a community that is better prepared to tackle its own problems and health interventions that will succeed because the community believes in them. Seeing the núcleo members come out to work month after month is strong evidence of the dedication of local people to improving their health. In Tevele, this has led to better protection from malaria, enhanced local knowledge about HIV prevention, the building of a basic health post, and the income-generating Zambo ni Zambo project described in Chapter 4.

The impact on the students was also significant. In the sandy yards of the homes they visited, they learned more about the social determinants of health than they ever could in a Canadian classroom. And unlike at the hospital in Massinga, where they saw only the sick and suffering, they met people at their best, at home where they are the experts. There they witnessed first-hand community strengths and weaknesses, and the role that income, education, housing, nutrition, and access to services play in deciding which families will thrive and which will suffer.

Democracy Diminished

These students also witnessed democracy – the rule of the people – at work, though in a form they had not seen before. The process of selecting priority concerns and the means of addressing them, led by those who are most affected by the decisions, is quite different from the democracy we experience at home. In Canada, the halls of power seem far removed from the challenges of everyday life and are often closed to the people who are most affected by political decisions. This generates disillusionment with the political process and cynicism about the individuals who seek election.

As a result, participation in elections at all levels is dwindling across Canada. This does not mean that people are no longer interested in public affairs. In my travels throughout the country, through politics, medicine, and my work with Upstream, I have been repeatedly impressed by the degree of knowledge, passion, and insight that Canadians have about important issues in their lives.

From big-picture issues such as international development and energy production to local concerns about the allocation of health care resources and community economic development, it's clear that people care deeply and want a say in the decisions that shape their lives and communities. The disconnect between passionate interest and lack of involvement stems from a growing perception that electoral politics are not a fruitful arena for public engagement. Be it the perception that governments are simply uninterested in their opinions, that they are beholden to large corporations, or that they are simply disinterested in the voice of the average citizen, people feel they are being ignored in the democratic process.

People sense that they are being ignored in the democratic process – that governments are simply uninterested in their opinions or that their hands are tied by international structures, beholden to large corporations.

Exacerbating this problem was Ottawa's decision in the late 1990s to replace the traditional door-to-door enumeration process with a permanent voter registry. The fact that voters are not actively registered with each election has intensified the decline in turnout and emphasized gaps in participation along social and economic lines. In 2011, the governing Saskatchewan Party attempted to make it harder to vote, with more stringent requirements for official identification, and to remove the ability of First Nations band offices and other organizations to attest to people's identities for voting purposes. This would have particularly affected on-reserve First Nations communities, leading to even lower turnout from groups that have traditionally been under-represented in elections. Fortunately, after a significant outcry from the general public, the media, and First Nations, the government backed down.

The issues of enumeration and voter turnout are extremely important, especially for the governments and political parties that rely on the mass participation of politically aware citizens rather than the support of well-heeled special interests. When citizens feel that their voices are heard, they are more likely to be involved as party members, activists, and candidates. This brings fresh energy and talent to the political process, increases voter turnout, and boosts the overall quality of debate.

No one understands local issues better than the people who live them every day. When decisions are made at a great distance, they lose the immediacy and common sense bred from this experience. In Saskatchewan, for example, there are more than a million people and at least that many ideas. There must be some way of bringing them forward and putting the best into practice.

What we need is less politics and more democracy. The only way to combat inequality and build a healthier society is through the meaningful participation of those who are most affected in the political process. A complementary system of distributed or participatory democracy would allow local people a more significant role in deciding their future. Rather than conflicting with our current parliamentary democracy, it would enrich it by helping counteract cynicism, increasing citizen involvement in government, and adding value to our representative democracy. Instead of bringing revolutionary change to our system of government, it would be an evolutionary process that reflects the ways in which – through population growth, mass literacy, and information sharing – society has changed, while preserving the foundations on which our democratic traditions are based.

Cotacachi

South America is home to one appealing model of such an evolutionary change. Cotacachi, a city in the foothills of the Ecuadorian Andes, has established citizen councils on education, health, the environment, democracy, and economic development. In these open councils, citizens from all walks of life identify key priorities and generate plans to address them. At the annual general council, they work together to determine how public resources will be distributed to meet these priorities.

The results of this participatory structure and process are proving to be remarkable. Infant mortality and illiteracy were identified as early priorities and are now all but eliminated. Electricity and sanitation services have been extended throughout the region. Perhaps the most important development is that citizens – rich and poor, Indigenous and European, men and women, young and old – are committed to working together to resolve issues. This model works because local and national governments support the process by following through with funding or changes to legislation based on the recommendations of the citizen councils. They also close the loop by communicating with the councils about which recommendations were followed, how this was done, and why.

The Cotacachi experience tells us that, given proper logistical supports and recognition from the existing structures of government, local areas can direct their own development. Of course, we cannot import wholesale a model from another context, but we can develop made-in-Canada versions of distributed democracy. For historical and geographical reasons, Saskatchewan has a strong tradition of community organization resulting in larger political changes. We have abundant natural resources and a small enough population to allow a high percentage of people to be personally involved. The development of flexible mechanisms, such as community assessment tools and staff and resource support for the organization of local councils, could provide the scaffolding for enhanced democratic decision making. This would then set the stage for a debate that moves from emphasizing tough, top-down direction to involving people in setting priorities, planning how to meet them, and working together to get results.

Indigenous Knowledge and Guidance

Inequality is when the government doesn't think you're worth the money.

— Cindy Blackstock, quoting a First Nations child,
Upstream Closing the Gap Conference[4]

Canada, like Ecuador, has a growing Indigenous population that has traditionally governed in a community-based and participatory fashion. The fastest-growing segment of Saskatchewan's population is Indigenous. Too often this is presented as a burden or a problem. I view it as our greatest opportunity. Having a young, vibrant population informed by proud tradition can make us the envy of other North American societies.

However, this opportunity is not without its challenges. If we return to the Canadian list of social determinants, one striking difference from other countries is the inclusion of Aboriginal status. This inclusion is controversial because it can be interpreted as suggesting that being First Nations, Métis, or Inuit is an inherent health risk. Health outcomes among Indigenous Canadians are worse in nearly every important measure of morbidity and mortality than among the non-Indigenous. However, when researchers control for factors such as income, education, employment, housing, and food security, these differences disappear.

The problem is that, in real life, these factors are too rarely controlled. As a result of the multi-generational effects of residential schools and other abuses and marginalizations, historical and ongoing, First Nations, Métis, and Inuit people are unequally and unduly burdened with poverty, lower levels of education, and an inordinate degree of incarceration. The result is an over-representation in ill health. Being Indigenous doesn't make you sicker – being Indigenous in Canada does.

A Healthy Society

Unless we work to change that gross inequality, that enormous and unsightly blight on our society, Aboriginal status will remain a useful shorthand for deprivation in the social determinants, and finding the best place for the coming generations will also remain a struggle. There is no quick remedy for these concerns. But there is an approach that is key, one supplied by the Truth and Reconciliation Commission of Canada.

Established in 2008 with a five-year mandate, the Truth and Reconciliation Commission travelled across the country, hosting hearings in which people who suffered as a result of the residential school system shared their stories. The commission's final report included ninety-four calls to action,[5] many of which illustrate the direct connection between Canada's colonial history and the current social determinants of health. Justice Murray Sinclair, who chaired the commission, put it this way: "We have described for you a mountain. We have shown you the path to the top. We call upon you to do the climbing."[6] The commission suggested actions to facilitate remembrance of and reconciliation for the residential schools, and described measures that could improve outcomes in child welfare, justice, education, language and culture, and health.

Taking our cues from the lived experiences of Indigenous people and respected leaders in their communities is a much-needed change in the nation-to-nation relationship. Too often in the past, experts have come from outside with answers that were simple, direct, and wrong, causing long-term harm to First Nations, Inuit, and Métis communities and damage to their traditional lands and way of life. Good money has been poured after bad ideas, and the result is no improvement in the communities and frustration on the part of the public. The answer to the problems faced by these communities lies in the communities themselves, in their strengths, their traditions, and their ideas and innovations.

Jordan River Anderson was from the Norway House Cree Nation.[7] Born with a rare muscular disorder, he needed hospital care for the first years of his life. Eventually, he was cleared to leave the hospital for a specialized foster care home in Winnipeg but required special home care services. The federal government and the Province of Manitoba disagreed regarding who should pay for this, and neither was willing to take on the expense. The stalemate dragged on for more than two years, during which Jordan's condition worsened. He died in hospital, never having seen his family home. Inspired by this story and the advocacy of First Nations groups, a private member's motion in support of Jordan's Principle was passed unanimously in the House of Commons in 2007. This established the expectation that, rather than seeking to avoid covering costs, the level of government that had first contact with a child would pay for the necessary services, and the final responsibility would be negotiated after the fact. According to the First Nations Child and Family Caring Society of Canada, "Jordan's Principle aims to make sure First Nations children can access all public services in a way that is reflective of their distinct cultural needs, takes full account of the historical disadvantage linked to colonization, and without experiencing any service denials, delays or disruptions related to their First Nations status."[8]

When I was working as part of the Advisory Group on Poverty Reduction to give recommendations for a poverty reduction strategy in Saskatchewan, this idea was very attractive to the public servants and community experts involved. I was impressed by how quickly and strongly the group developed a principle that services should be delivered across the province regardless of jurisdiction.[9] This runs counter to a long-standing reality in Canada, in which First Nations reserves are like islands where services that are provided to most Canadians are simply non-existent. In terms of their coverage in health, education, child welfare, and more, the provinces resemble Swiss cheese, and the results for people are starkly different, depending on where they live. For example, half of status First Nations children in Canada live in poverty, with Saskatchewan and Manitoba sharing the shame of on-reserve poverty rates at over 60 percent.[10]

Unfortunately, the implementation of Jordan's Principle has mostly been limited to a narrow interpretation of health services, and even this has been resisted in court. As a result, First Nations children fare far worse than other children in Canada when it comes to the delivery of health, education, recreation, and child welfare services.[11] One of the Truth and Reconciliation Commission's recommendations was to "call upon all levels of government to fully implement Jordan's Principle."

Cindy Blackstock of the First Nations Child and Family Caring Society of Canada has been a key voice for justice for First Nations children for more than a decade. She led a complaint to the Canadian Human Rights Tribunal, claiming that the government's failure to provide services on the same terms to all children amounted to discrimination. In its January 2016 decision regarding the case, the tribunal found the Government of Canada to be discriminating against First Nations children on the basis of race and ethnic origin and ordered Ottawa to rectify the situation and to apply Jordan's Principle by providing culturally appropriate and equitable child welfare services.[12] The government is fighting the decision in court, but with the tireless advocacy of Blackstock and her supporters, this idea holds the promise of a better, fairer life for Canadian children.

Healing the wounds of colonization, past and present, means refusing to let jurisdictional boundaries or ethnicity serve as excuses for maintaining injustice. It means going beyond narrow interpretations of the duty to consult to forging real partnerships. It means exploring innovative and controversial strategies, such as resource revenue sharing and other means of honouring treaty rights and addressing persistent inequalities. It means working with leaders and community members to develop governance models and accountabilities that will make those innovative strategies successful. And it means working together to communicate clearly to Canadians, Indigenous and non-Indigenous, that ending inequality is of the highest national priority.

The only way to work toward a better future for Indigenous people in Canada is to work alongside them. Communities are better than any outside agency at identifying their own needs and can also identify the solutions that will work for them. There will be no easy fix. Patient investment and the development of long-term relationships built on mutual respect are both necessary. Given the attention it deserves, however, this process will contribute to the long-term health and prosperity of the entire country.

As long as Canada is a nation divided, it cannot truly develop. When we finally recognize that all peoples have made a valuable contribution to this country, particularly those long neglected and marginalized, only then will we be on our way to building a healthy society.

Life of the Party

Political parties, the current vehicles for direct citizen involvement in politics, are often closed to real change. It takes a moment of crisis to galvanize the necessary soul searching to make bold decisions. The rest of the time, parties are too concerned with electoral success, with appearing reasonable and electable to a skeptical public, to entertain truly novel ideas. The product of this inertia is the great divide between the converted few and the general public, with a wide distance between the ideas needed for a healthy society and the political will to achieve them.

By introducing a means for more direct citizen involvement, we can build a bridge between communities, social movements, and electoral politics. Despite the criticism of the way in which parties operate, they are the most likely vehicle for this kind of experimentation. Let's take, for example, the case of the Saskatchewan New Democratic Party, the one with which I'm most familiar. Recently, it has undergone a major change. After governing from 1991 under Premiers Roy Romanow and Lorne Calvert, the NDP was defeated in 2007 by the Saskatchewan Party (a right-of-centre coalition of disaffected Liberals and rebranded Progressive Conservatives). Its ranks were thinned to twenty members of the Legislative Assembly. In the 2011 election, the Saskatchewan Party won a strengthened majority, with the NDP losing eleven more seats, including that of the party leader in what had traditionally been a stronghold. A similar result in 2016 saw the new leader lose his seat and an even greater majority for the Sask Party. What has often been referred to as the "natural governing party" of Saskatchewan has been reduced to a shadow of its former strength. This should give it both cause and room to reconsider itself deeply, a unique opportunity to experiment with democracy. At various times in the past, the party has made attempts to renew itself, some more successful than others (such as the famous New Deal for People, under Allan Blakeney). The common flaw, however, has been the focus on a review or renewal effort, an exercise lasting a fixed amount of time. When the party flounders and extinction seems imminent, efforts are made at resuscitation, but once it regains enough strength to win another election, its health is neglected and the cycle repeats itself.

What is needed is a process by which healthy debate is maintained, where renewal is ongoing rather than periodic and cosmetic.

A democracy is not a fixed and perfect system. Constant reconsideration is required to ensure that it functions smoothly and is truly representative. For a political party, this means a continuous process of citizen engagement to keep it active and healthy, one that goes beyond selling memberships and passing resolutions at conventions. Consultation can't be token and inconsistent; it must be constant and meaningful. A party that makes a point of heeding the diverse opinions of multiple and varied constituencies can set a vision for change at a larger level. Structures that enforce accountability of its leadership to the party membership will strengthen the commitment of citizens to that vision. This could result in the foundation of functional local councils on key issues, such as the economy, education, the environment, and health care, which is to say a meaningful system of citizen leadership in addressing the determinants of health. In this way, Canada could follow the example of other countries that have made significant reforms and increased citizen engagement. Local areas, armed with local understanding and expertise, can work with provincial and federal governments to direct their own development. The party that leads such a transformation would be a party that had truly found its voice: the voice of one who listens.

A Question of Trust

The role and influence of money in Canadian politics have received much attention during recent years. Cash-for-access events, where people buy an expensive ticket to spend time with key decision-makers, have come under scrutiny at the federal and provincial level. The link between which companies donate and which companies benefit most from government policies and contracts is increasingly visible. The growing perception that wealthy donors have an outsized influence on federal and provincial leaders has prompted six provinces to ban or limit corporate and union donations to political parties.

The fact is, when we talk about the problems with political donations, we're not really talking about campaign financing. We're talking about something much more fundamental. We're talking about trust. We're talking about how the public views political leaders. Can they be trusted to do the right thing? Can we trust them to be objective in their interactions with companies? Will they make the best decisions for the people who elected them, rather than for companies seeking favourable laws and contracts?

Political parties need donations to maintain an organization, promote their message, and run election campaigns, but where that money comes from and how it is raised matters a great deal. The primary goal of a party and its representatives cannot be to help their donors. It must be to achieve the best for the people. As well as providing guidance on the best ways to measure the success of policy choices, the health field offers us some important insights on this question of trust.

In the field of medicine, there's a long-standing practice whereby pharmaceutical companies give gifts to physicians. Sometimes, these are simple things, such as pens, mugs, or notepads, all emblazoned with the company name and logo. Or they can be bigger and more costly: a golf trip, a fancy dinner. They can even consist of direct payments to physicians who enroll their patients in a drug study. The greater the degree of connection, the more expensive the gift, the greater the influence. But the gift doesn't have to be large. Research shows that even the smallest tokens – a pen, a pad of paper, an anatomy poster – influence behaviour.[13] The pharmaceutical companies aren't giving mugs to doctors because they want them to have a good hot cup of coffee. It's because they want them to prescribe their drugs.

As Dr. David Grande said in a 2010 article in the *Journal of General Internal Medicine*, "Gifts associated with pharmaceutical detailing are motivated by a single goal – to increase the sales of a company's products."[14] The same is true for corporate gifts to political parties. The big donors who give tens of thousands of dollars aren't doing it solely because they believe in the party's vision. They're giving large sums because they believe it will pay off, that it will influence the government's thinking and behaviour. These are not gifts: they're investments.

In recent years, medical associations have tried to decrease the influence of pharmaceutical companies through gifts. In my own practice, I've avoided taking gifts or meeting with pharmaceutical salespeople.

These efforts to diminish influence are occurring in one of the most trusted professions. The public consistently ranks physicians in the company of such trusted groups as pharmacists and firemen. Sixty-five percent of Canadians trust doctors. Only 6 percent trust politicians.[15] Physicians realize that trust is their greatest asset, with both the public and their patients. If we want our patients to take our advice and change their behaviour, we need to have their solid trust.

Our elected representatives should also want to be trusted as a profession. For the good of the democratic process, the public needs to know that its voice has the most clout, and corporate donations impede that confidence. Even if some perfect barrier preventing the influence of donors could be established, the public would still believe that it remains powerful. Whatever the reality, the perception is clear. People don't trust the political profession and they don't trust it for some very clear reasons.

What are those reasons? In Saskatchewan, for example, political parties have received some questionable donations.[16] Public institutions – universities, libraries, and municipal governments – are making donations, as are out-of-province corporations. At big gala dinners, people pay extra to have access to members of the government. Until a few months ago, regular top-ups of the premier's salary of nearly half a million dollars in the last decade were directly connected to donations. The public knows this, and they are not impressed.[17] Eighty-one percent of Saskatchewan people believe that no public institution should contribute to a political party; 69 percent oppose out-of-province donations; and 74 percent feel that no donation money should come from charities. When elected officials insist that accepting financial contributions is perfectly fine, their reputations are damaged, as are those of all legislators. When people look at politicians and believe they are working for money and power, it cheapens work that is absolutely crucial.

We need to kick this drug. We need to get our political process out from under the influence. In response to mounting criticism of cash-for-access and other dubious practices, jurisdictions across Canada have been limiting corporate and union donations.[18] Having transparent rules that limit outside influence keeps voters and their interests at the centre of elections and governance. Healthy democracies put people at the heart of the political process. This is how trust in politics, in what should be a noble profession, can be rebuilt. But that's only a part of it. No one can trust someone who doesn't trust them in return. The bigger step is reinvesting in democracy, in demonstrating that we actually believe that the people have the wisdom to lead.

Leaping across the Divide

Truly reviving democracy requires a leap of faith. We must trust ourselves and our neighbours. We must trust that, given the opportunity, we, the people, will choose what is best for us. The people can, given the opportunity, take the lead in building a healthier society. The challenge before us is to create the mechanisms to let those ideas be heard and put into action.

Such a leap of faith requires trust, a commodity that is unfortunately in short supply in the current political climate. For many people – people who would call themselves proponents of democracy – the first response to such ideas is fear. They think that if ordinary folks become too involved in decision making, democracy will be co-opted by right- or left-wing radicals. The only way to get people to trust you is to trust them. It's also the best way to help someone become trustworthy. It's risky, which is hard to accept in uncertain times, but the frame of reference of the determinants of health offers us some hope. It provides a standard to strive for, based on common values. This type of framing is not intended to deceive and control. Rather, its point is to stop the ongoing manipulation and fragmentation that characterize our interactions. The intent is to reorient our public discourse to the honest identification of common goals and the means to reach them. The common goal of a healthy society can be a means of bridging divides between people who initially seem irreconcilable.

Take, for a moment, the language of freedom. Enemies of the concept of the state, who believe that government is a curse, often invoke freedom to advance their views: freedom from taxation, from regulation, from responsibility for the failures of foolish others. This freedom is like that of the adolescent who wants to enjoy the benefits of parental support without curfew or chores. The child's parents, on the other hand, have chosen to bind themselves to one another and to their offspring, to support them and love them. Through this bond, they have traded immature freedom, which is selfish and hollow, for deeper freedom: the freedom to love each other fully, to embrace the challenges of raising children, to accept joyously the responsibilities accompanying their expanded rights. This view of freedom is also the attitude of mature citizenship, a citizenship that recognizes the great freedom that is represented by universal health care, unemployment insurance, secure pensions, and a fair and compassionate justice system. The mature citizen asks the ancient question of Cain, "Am I my brother's keeper?" and replies, "Hell, yes, and happier for it!" He knows that his contribution, which is needed by his neighbour now, not only does that neighbour good but also bolsters a system that will support him in his own time of need, which comes for most. The next step in that freedom is not simply accepting and contributing to the common good, but becoming involved in its development. Populist movements, like the Tea Party in the United States, though often misdirected in their anger, have this at their heart. Ordinary people feel, correctly, that their interests and voices are ignored in the decision-making processes of so-called democracies. Honest intentions and frustrations are diverted from meaningful expression to angry demonstrations. There is a temptation, when faced with adversaries who appear illogical and intransigent, to override them with force or ignore them and proceed through trickery. The way back from culture wars, from the divisive and negative, is not less democracy. It is more: it is deeper and more open debate, it is the consideration of profound and complex notions, and it is the constant revisiting of core goals.

In the example above, what initially appears to be a right-left issue becomes far more nuanced upon further exploration. This is a useful exercise, because though the right-left split can be real, it can also be misrepresented and exaggerated. For my own understanding of left and right wing, I find it helpful and instructive to boil the difference down to two clear definitions. In essence, right-wing philosophy can be described as "every man for himself" and left-wing as "we're all in this together." This is an over-simplification, of course, but it's useful to get back to first principles, untainted by words such as "capitalism" and "socialism," words that have been misrepresented and misused by opponents and proponents alike.

Advancing to a subtler description, we might say that the left emphasizes bringing out the best for all of society, whereas the right concentrates on bringing out the best in ourselves. At its best, the right encourages individual responsibility and initiative. At its worst, it blames and abandons the poor, and breeds judgment and scorn for the less fortunate. The left, at its best, supports those who are most in need and seeks to distribute the good of society equitably. At its worst, it fosters victimhood, mediocrity, and sloth. To paraphrase Gandhi, there can be no system that removes the necessity for people to be good. At times the far left is guilty of trying to do just that, of legislating utopia. For its part, the far right chases a utopia of false freedom – freedom from any responsibility to our fellow humans – abandoning the systems that allow people to develop enough to make wise moral decisions.

A view that incorporates the best of these two political philosophies is that we need to create the conditions for everyone to maintain a reasonable standard of living while also providing opportunities for people to make good choices. We need to take care of the social needs of the population without losing sight of the fact that a well-functioning economy is a necessity for that well-being. The reason I choose to align myself on what's described as the left of the political spectrum is that while an attitude of "we're all in this together" allows room to emphasize an ethic of personal responsibility and initiative, an attitude of "every man for himself" cannot provide for everyone and actively interferes with an organized approach to improving society. The key to a healthier society is not the elimination of government; it is the restructuring of government to be what it should be: a mechanism for achieving the will of the people, a truly democratic institution that allows the good instincts and ideas of people to be reflected in a larger plan. It is the idea of society as a project that all of us are working on and government as the people's workshop.

Father Figuring

For a long time, my personal motto has been "be right-wing with yourself and left-wing with everyone else." That is, be demanding of myself, insisting on hard work and moral rectitude, while accepting the weaknesses of others. With time, and what I hope to be some maturity, I've come to be more comfortable with my own weaknesses and failures, realizing that beating myself up for each moment of laziness or moral miscue is exhausting and counter-productive. I've also come to understand – in life and in medical practice – that there are times when, for the good of the other, one must demand that he or she shows strength and resolve. Sometimes you need to refrain from helping people so that they can help themselves.

All this is to say that, though I've arrived, conscious and committed, at what could be described as a left position in our current spectrum, that spectrum is broad. It is a practical idealism, a search to do the good that works. Similar to the tool box approach to economic policy, it allows flexibility and the capacity to recognize the ideals behind the positions of those on the "other side." The goal of creating a healthy society is helpful in escaping the most simplistic left-right dichotomy. Its focus is on outcomes, on the best results for people. The methods need to be analyzed for what will achieve those outcomes, but that's the metric, not whether they pass an ideological purity test.

All too often, we assume that people who disagree with us have the worst of motivations. Not only is this a shallow analysis, it also eliminates the possibility of finding common ground. Recognizing that the intentions of our opponents are valid even though we might not agree with them allows us to move beyond hyper-partisan polarization in search of a common good.

My own approach to this is informed by my relationship with my father. As I wrote this book, I often thought about how he would react to the ideas within. Wally Meili has been a card-carrying member of the Saskatchewan Party. His political affiliation has always been to the right, and for as long as I can remember, to the right of mine (I recall him describing me to a friend at eight or nine as "a good kid but a bit left-wing"). He worked for Progressive Conservative Saskatchewan premier Grant Devine in the 1980s, investigating alternative markets for Saskatchewan agricultural products. His brother Ernie ran for a Reform Party nomination in Saskatoon during the 1990s. When we talk politics, we frequently butt heads over parties, policies, and personalities.

If I didn't know him, I might see him as an adversary, someone misguided and wrong. But I know better; he is a very good man. I've never met anyone who doesn't like Wally. He's generous, kind, and genuinely interested in people. He's been the model, throughout my life, of the good Samaritan, always helping people out of small jams and big problems. He's well read and well travelled, a successful farmer, and a dedicated dad and grandpa. In recent years, he's become a philanthropist, bringing medical supplies to aid projects in Central America and organizing clean water systems for Haiti. Beyond politics, we have a lot in common (sometimes too much; I frequently find myself sounding exactly like him, especially now that I have my own kids).

So, when we disagree politically, we have to be careful. We can't discard each other's opinions, can't simply walk away and dismiss the other as a fool. Coming from a place of mutual respect, we seek out common ground, and our discussions about the determinants of health have made sense to him. I don't think he'll ever be a social democrat (though one of my great accomplishments in life was seeing him join the NDP so that he could vote for his son in the leadership race), but he reminds me that the "other side" is often not as other as it seems.

Eddies and Loops

It's important to remember that we need to look beyond our normal political circles and engage with those whose opinions differ from our own, as – paradoxically, in these days of social media – it's very easy to become isolated. My experience of the 2011 federal election is a great example. In Saskatchewan, two NDP candidates had reasonable chances of unseating Conservative MPs Nettie Wiebe in Saskatoon–Rosetown–Biggar and Noah Evanchuk in Moose Jaw-Palliser. As expected, these races turned out to be very close, with the incumbent Conservatives keeping their seats by less than 3 percent of the vote. But if you'd consulted my Facebook feed beforehand, you'd have thought that the NDP would romp to victory. Nearly everyone's profile picture showed an Orange Crush can, and status updates were full of links to stories by NDP organizers or in sympathetic newspapers. This occurred partly because more of my friends vote NDP than don't but also because

Facebook and other social media sites track what you read and then show you more of the same. Rather than expanding their awareness of what's happening in the world, users become more entrenched in their own beliefs.

With that kind of positive affirmation loop, people can become smug, assuming that any thinking person sees the world as they do and dismissing anyone who disagrees with them. Rather than helping them to reach their goals and serve their cause, the social network isolates them among a twinkle of activists, leading them to conclude that they're winning when they're merely hearing the echo of their own opinions. This isn't to say that the use of social media is terrible, just that they have their limitations and are no replacement for conversations.

For the good of all people, not just those on our list of friends, we need to take the conversation beyond local loops to include a wider audience. The way to do this is, first, to return to the language of health, language that works across divides of right and left, and then to take the conversation everywhere: to churches and classrooms, union halls and company boardrooms. We need to risk ridicule on right-wing talk radio, not just stick to the CBC. This has to be genuine – a real discussion with people, regardless of their affiliations. The purpose is not to convince the world of one set of solutions; to find common ground, we must recognize that no one has a monopoly on wisdom. If I disregard the opinion of someone who opposes me, then I am the fool.

The High Road Is Hard to Find

To many who've been through the hard slog of working for change, be it in the political arena or civil society, this all sounds pretty naïve. There are people in this game, whether on the other side or, even more dangerously, among your own allies, who will do and say things that are dishonest, mean-spirited, and manipulative. There's no getting around that. But there may be a way to get above it, which is to get over it. I say from experience that the more you take the bait, the more you worry about who's saying what behind your back, the more you risk getting sucked into the worst of the game. It doesn't have to be that way. If you can avoid descending into accusations and negativity about your opponents, if you can avoid mentioning them at all and stick to talking about ideas, then there is room for a different kind of politics.

People are frustrated by what they see in electoral politics. They see complex issues being dumbed down and misrepresented. They see childish bickering. They see scandal. They see politicians who are more worried about optics than vision, chasing polls rather than saying what they truly believe. They see growing division and self-interest replacing a sense of common good. At a time when more people care about the issues that matter, they are becoming cynical and apathetic about the process. Talented men and women who could be great candidates, who could lead the way to meaningful change, are scared off by the behaviour of their potential colleagues and opponents. Many people are either withdrawing completely or contenting themselves with working for change on the margins while the mainstream gets polluted.

What I believe, and what drove me to seek public office, is that the time is right for positive politics. The demand is growing for something better from our public representatives. There is an appetite for a different approach, for candidates who are thoughtful and principled, who speak with sincerity, with genuine humour. There is a desire for what Calgary mayor Naheed Nenshi called "Politics in full sentences."[19] People want someone who can communicate with them about complicated political issues in a way that respects their intelligence, someone who doesn't dumb things down, but translates the issues into core concepts on which we can build.

Right now, the low road is congested. Attack ads, scandal mongering, and behind-the-scenes manipulation are the apparent tools of the trade. Each party decries the dirty tricks of the others but excuses itself when it resorts to the same tactics, pointing out the mote in their brother's eye and ignoring the log in their own. In such an atmosphere, taking the high road isn't easy. But it becomes easier when ideas, notions of equality and justice – the ideas of a healthy society – are what drive people to get involved. And it can work; it's where there is room for growth. The space is on the high road. The space is in appealing to the best in people, to hope and to dignity, to the forgotten notion that we really are all in this together. Imagine for a moment a political party that has a plan to build a healthier society, a plan based on addressing the determinants of health.

Imagine a party with an open code of conduct for its own behaviour, regardless of what the other side might do. Imagine a party that, when in opposition, avoids cheap, partisan bickering but refers constantly to the stories of real people and the issues that affect them. Imagine a platform that outlines the changes to be made in each of the key determinants. Then imagine a government that involves the people meaningfully in decision making, judging every decision not on short-term political gains but on the real impact on people's health. Imagine, instead of spin and opportunistic funding announcements, clear communication on the reasoning behind decisions, and elections that are truly based on whether or not the country has become a healthier place. This is a far cry from what we see now, but there is room and appetite for such an approach. Taking the high road is not only the good and noble thing to do; it's also what will win people's confidence. If there is enough pressure to create a more equal, healthier society, candidates will emerge who speak this language. Our democratic system is suffering, and the remedy is not harder fought, more polarized politics. What is needed to build a healthy society is deeper democracy.

12

OUR FUTURE TOGETHER

The impact of determinants of health and lifestyle choices is well known to governments and to health care organizations. Unfortunately, the key problem lies in turning this understanding into concrete actions that have an impact on individual Canadians and communities.

– Commission on the Future of Health Care in Canada, *Building on Values*[1]

Another way to strengthen the social determinants of health is to support candidates of political parties that are receptive to the social determinants of health concept. Candidates who favour these ideas and the public policies that flow from them should be supported, and those that currently do not need to be pressured to adopt these positions.

– Juha Mikkonen and Dennis Raphael, "Social Determinants of Health"[2]

True prosperity comes from using the best of our abilities in economic and social policy to achieve the health and well-being of all people, rather than exhausting that health and well-being in the exclusive pursuit of economic wealth. Understanding how social determinants influence health outcomes at individual and population levels gives us a framework through which decisions can be made and measured. Because countries with greater equality do better in both social and physical measures of health, we have a general direction for how to proceed. Sharing public resources equitably to improve the health of everyone is just and compassionate. It also increases economic productivity, public safety, and the quality of life for everyone, from the poor to the rich. It's the right thing and the smart thing to do.

Throughout this book, I've explored some of the key determinants in detail, through the lens of real people and real policy options. This is an example of how a health filter, informed by the best local and imported sources of evidence, can guide political decision making. Perhaps more importantly, this focus can help us to realign our democratic processes toward a shared notion, an identifiable common good. People care about health. They care about their own health and the health of their family. They also care about the health of society.

The core idea of this book is not just that health should guide our policy decisions: it should be the language of our politics. Because people care about health, they are likely to respond to political messages that reflect that concern. This is about framing – not in a manipulative way, but in a way that connects diverse and complex issues to a common concern. The point is not to advance the marketing success of one party – it's a means of rehabilitating a sick political system. A focus on health, which an increasingly aware population is demanding, can force every party to reconsider its decisions and positions in relation to the determinants. It can establish an environment in which, rather than being bombarded shoppers in the marketplace of clashing ideas and conflicting priorities, people can see themselves as part of a shared project, as working together toward the goal of a healthier society.

Clinical Trials

In the spring of 2017, my practice changed drastically. I still do occasional family medicine shifts to keep up my skills and to stay connected with the patients whose lives and stories inspire me, but that's not where

I spend most of my time. Encouraged by Rudolf Virchow's idea of politics as medicine on a larger scale, I ran in a by-election and was elected as the MLA for Saskatoon Meewasin as part of the Opposition New Democratic caucus. Meewasin is a fascinating constituency, with inner-city, high-density downtown apartments, older heritage neighbourhoods, and new suburbs. The word "Meewasin" is Cree and is usually translated as "beautiful," an appropriate name for an area that runs along the South Saskatchewan River. After I was elected, one of the Indigenous studies professors at the university told me that the word also means "good." I try to keep that in mind as a reminder that the purpose of our elected officials is to work for the good, what is good for us all.

This by-election was not my first effort. I had run for leadership of the Saskatchewan NDP in 2009 and 2013. In both of these contests, the theme was that of building a healthy society, and the social determinants of health concepts informed the platform. Given that I was relatively unknown and had never held elected office, this message was remarkably well received, and I finished second on both occasions, in 2013 by a nail-bitingly, heartbreakingly narrow margin of forty-four votes. After the first race (along with continuing my clinical and academic work), I wrote the first edition of this book, clarifying the ideas that had inspired me to run, and I continued to work as a volunteer on provincial and federal campaigns. After the second, along with many of the people who had been part of the campaign team, I helped found Upstream to give these ideas a national platform.

In 2016, the Saskatchewan Party won another massive majority, and for the second straight election, the leader of the NDP lost his seat. As a result, there will be another leadership contest in 2018, the third for the provincial NDP since it lost power in 2007. Given the near misses of the last efforts and the need for a credible alternative, a healthy choice, I've chosen to put my name back in the proverbial hat.

There's a parallel here with an earlier phase of my life. When I first applied to medical school, I told the admissions committee that I wanted to work with underserved populations, particularly in the developing world. The committee members asked where I'd been and what I'd done in that field so far. Truth was, though I'd read and thought a great deal, I was a twenty-one-year-old kid from the farm with no experience outside the country. Needless to say, they thought I was a bit naïve, and they were right. I sought to remedy that, taking a year off from university to spend several months in South America, volunteering and learning how to work respectfully alongside people from another culture.

I returned and applied a second time, this time coming closer as I made the waiting list. I enrolled for another year of school, studying even harder than before and improving my grades. I also organized a special project that took prosthetic limbs from Canada to land mine victims in Nicaragua. I applied a third time, and the interview committee was much more confident that my experiences had prepared me to study and practise medicine. Whether things would have turned out as well if I'd been accepted immediately, I'll never know, but the trials of getting in gave me great learning experiences that simply strengthened my determination and dedication.

Upon hearing that I was running again for the NDP leadership, a lot of people brought out the "third time's the charm" line. That's a nice notion, but if this works, there won't be anything magical about it. Persistence and hard work, and lessons learned through mistakes and lucky guesses, are the ingredients for success in repeat efforts. At the heart of it all, however, is the question of whether this idea of a healthy society does what I believe it can. By reaching across political lines to a deeper shared value of health, and using that framing to bring forward ideas that inspire, we can unite people in a common cause.

The surprising near wins from my first efforts gave me hope, as has the growth of Upstream as a respected national voice. It's also been interesting to see this message popping up in the materials of other political figures and parties. The federal NDP was the first party in Canada to showcase the social determinants, in a policy statement titled "Prevention Is Better Than Cure" that was released during the lead-up to the 2015 federal election. When Steve Kent ran for the leadership of the Progressive Conservatives of Newfoundland and Labrador, he had a social determinants focus and advocated for Health in All Policies. He wasn't elected leader, but he later served as minister of health and started the process of bringing in Health in All Policies that is being continued by the current Liberal government. And Jane Philpott, the federal health minister, has described her own path of being inspired by Virchow's quote and her experiences of working with marginalized populations as the impetus for her move from family medicine to politics.

However, we have yet to see a major party run a major campaign with this framing, with achieving the well-being of the public as the primary purpose of its politics. Should I be successful in the upcoming leadership race and in bringing these ideas into the platform for the next provincial election, it's a remarkable opportunity to try this promising new approach. Even more exciting is the prospect of, having won the election, working with the people of Saskatchewan to design and implement policies that reflect this shared preoccupation with health and that result in real improvements in the quality of our lives.

Shovels in the Ground

My venture in trying out this theme in a leadership campaign pales in comparison with another social determinants success story. Despite the setback when the provincial government rescinded funding for Station 20 West, the community-based organizations behind the project regrouped, redesigned, and continued to fundraise. The politics of their decision and the need to downsize meant that the dental clinic, SWITCH, and the West Side Community Clinic would no longer be involved; the presence of some of the other intended partners was at risk, and the eco-friendly status of the building would have to be downgraded. Nonetheless, spurred on by the success of a Friends of Station 20 West Facebook group that garnered thousands of members in the days following the announcement of the loss of funding, along with a tremendous show of support at a community rally, the organizers committed to raising the necessary money to start construction of the more modest version of the original plan. Volunteers put on dozens of fundraisers, distributed change jars to area businesses, and held bake sales and buy-a-brick sponsorship campaigns. The City of Saskatoon sold the land to the project for a dollar, and early support came in the form of donations and mortgage guarantees from public-sector unions and a local credit union. At the end of 2010, ten Christian church communities committed to raising funds within their congregations during the

Christmas season in support of Station 20 West's Good Food Junction grocery store.

The Station 20 West board had learned of the loss of government funding on the Easter weekend of 2008. After three years of struggle, with prospects for success sometimes looking very dim, the board learned of a large donation from Saskatoon philanthropist Joe Remai on Easter weekend, 2011. With another substantial donation from the Kinsmen Foundation of Saskatoon shortly afterward, enough money had been raised to start construction. Accompanied by a troupe of older activists called the Raging Grannies singing "Shovels in the Ground" (to the tune of "Bringing in the Sheaves"), dozens of community members and supporters came out to celebrate the successful campaign and applaud a ceremonial sod turning on a rainy day in July 2011. Station 20 West opened its doors in September 2012.

Some of its original elements were missed. I certainly wished that our clinic had remained part of Station 20 West. There are still many possibilities to work together in addressing the determinants of health, but they're much more likely to happen when everyone is in the same building. The traffic of patients through the building would also have helped other co-locators to become well known. But the fact is, Station 20 West didn't happen according to plan, and there have been other setbacks, including the closing of the Good Food Junction, which for various reasons couldn't make enough money to keep going. However, though the initial vision did not become a reality, in some ways what happened is the better story. The people of Saskatoon are now more familiar with the issues of food insecurity and housing shortages in the city's core. People on both sides of this often divided town came together, first in reaction to the government's bad decision but then in action for change. The result is a project that not only serves the people of the core, but will also stand as an emblem of solidarity, a true community victory.

Today, Station 20 West is a vibrant place where the community can come together and try new things. Some of these will be short-lived, but others will flourish and grow into local institutions. The current co-locators include the Quint Development Corporation, CHEP Good Food, a public health outreach centre from the Saskatoon Health Region, early childhood development programming, a university outreach centre, and a locally run cafe. It's also become an essential community centre, with hundreds of groups using it for meetings. In fact, the first Idle No More meeting was held at Station 20 West, kicking off the national Indigenous movement that electrified Canada in 2012–13 and continues to advocate for justice for Indigenous people. As a community centre that addresses the social determinants of health, Station 20 West is part of a network of exemplary projects across Canada that manifest as practical collaborations to address the health needs of local communities.

Escaping from the Phantom Zone

These successes show that ideas of the determinants of health can have currency with the public. This is supported by the work of the Saskatoon researchers who first identified the extent of the health disparities between low-income neighbourhoods and the rest of the city. After that initial research but prior to the release of their evidence-based recommendations to resolve the problem, they conducted a study of community opinions.[3] They started by phoning five thousand Saskatoon residents, male and female, Indigenous and non-Indigenous, from wealthy and poor neighbourhoods. The participants were asked to give their opinions regarding which factors determined health, the relationship between income and certain conditions and behaviours, interventions that would make a difference, and the acceptable level of health disparity.

The results of this study were largely encouraging. Though people somewhat over-emphasized the role of nutritious food and exercise compared with other determinants, they generally recognized that income, education, employment, and other social circumstances have an impact on health outcomes. They tended not to realize just how much income influenced the likelihood of developing certain health conditions or of engaging in harmful behaviours such as substance abuse or smoking.

Though many respondents did not fully understand the role of the determinants of health, they did voice a strong preference for more equal health outcomes. Most who expressed an opinion said that there should be no or very little difference in health outcomes based on income. There was no support for the huge inequalities that exist today. Perhaps more encouraging yet, not only did people believe that the current inequality in health outcomes was unacceptable, they were also overwhelmingly (83 percent) convinced that something could be done about it.

So what we have is a situation where people have a reasonable understanding, to a degree, of the role of played by the social determinants of health, believe that large inequalities in health outcomes are unacceptable, and think that something can and should be done about them. However, despite this understanding and concern, the topic receives little attention in the present discourse on public policy. York University professor Dennis Raphael, a prominent author in the field of health determinants, suggests that they have been consigned to a Superman II–esque Phantom Zone – powerful and important, but out of sight and out of mind. He explains, "Canadian research and advocacy activities in the service of strengthening the SDOH [social determinants of health] are so divorced from everyday public policy activity, media discourse and public awareness as to metaphorically suggest that SDOH researchers and advocates exist in a Phantom Zone of irrelevance."[4] He urges advocates of public health to make the noise necessary to draw attention to this important issue.

Interestingly, the Phantom Zone idea prompted a surprising critique of the first edition of this book. In the summer of 2013, I was in Yellowknife for the annual meeting of the Canadian Medical Association (CMA), on behalf of Canadian Doctors for Medicare. As a professional association that represents doctors, the CMA has often been seen – fairly or unfairly – as working primarily for their interests, with patients and health equity sometimes seeming to be an afterthought. This impression was particularly strong during the presidencies of Brian Day (2007–08) and Robert Ouellet (2008–09), both vocal advocates for privatization (and owners of private, for-profit health care facilities) who used their tenure to call for greater private payment for essential health services.

As I had come to view the organization with a degree of distrust, the Yellowknife meeting was like stepping into – to continue with the Superman references – a Bizarro CMA. The keynote speaker was Michael Marmot, who presented the challenging message that "inequality is killing on a grand scale" and asserted that governments, and physicians, must address the causes of health inequities. This concept has been getting greater attention through the CMA presidencies of Ontario's Jeff Turnbull, Newfoundland's John Haggie, Yellowknife's Anna Reid, Edmonton's Louis Francescutti, and Kingston's Chris Simpson. The attention of the CMA to the social determinants was taken further with the CMA's 2013 release of "Health Care in Canada: What Makes Us Sick?"[5] The result of a series of town halls across Canada, this report underlined the degree to which four key determinants – income, housing, early childhood development, and food security – influence the health and well-being of Canadians and offered a dozen recommendations on how to deal with them. These include important general ideas about tackling poverty, substandard housing, food insecurity, and the poor health of Indigenous people. They also propose more specific changes, such as pharmacare, Housing First initiatives, and basic income: ideas that could be considered quite radical in today's political context. Yet here they are, emanating from what is seen as one of the most conservative professional organizations in the country. Why? Because whatever self-interest may influence the politics of physicians, the purpose of the profession is still, at its heart, to achieve the best health outcomes for patients.

In Yellowknife, Michael Marmot was kind enough to offer a few words of introduction at the local launch of *A Healthy Society*. I was honoured that he had read the book and a little bit star-struck that he was willing to stand with me beside the children's section in the Yellowknife Book Cellar and discuss ideas with a small group of interested doctors and community members. He did, however, take umbrage with my reference to the social determinants as languishing in a Phantom Zone. Stating that this disconnect no longer applied, he cited the CMA meeting as an example that these concepts were becoming mainstream and that the public was ready for them to influence policy.

I hope he's right, and I think that the CMA's 2013 town hall report, the success of Upstream, and the growing use of social determinants language in various political and issue campaigns do suggest we're finally breaking out of the Phantom Zone. However, inequality continues to deepen in Canada, many cities still experience housing and homelessness crises, food insecurity remains a chronic problem, especially among First

Nations and Métis people, and early childhood development programs are inconsistent and inadequate across the country.

A great deal of work must be done to make sure our recognition of the role of social factors in determining health outcomes translates into action that improves the lives of Canadians. And what Dennis Raphael and other researchers recognize is that, if this concept were more widely understood, and people were aware of its power, then it could have a huge impact on politics, on public policy in economics, education, environment, and ultimately on the most meaningful outcome: the health of our society and the people who constitute its fabric.

Part of my job as a family doctor is to present complex issues in language that people can understand. There is a pressing need to do just that with the social determinants of health – to put them into context and to clarify them so that people can perceive how relevant they are to their own lives. The dual purpose of this book is to highlight the need to share these ideas and to serve as a tool for doing so. Hopefully, the stories recounted here can bring this issue home for readers and spur them to action.

Often when people want to create change, they focus on what is wrong with the current situation. I've certainly done that myself and still do to some degree in this book. Pointing out flaws is easy and can be a useful first step, but in and of itself, it won't produce change. In fact, a list of woes that lacks a set of solutions can be paralyzing, leading people to conclude that problems are too dire to fix. In the previous chapters, I discussed a few interventions that could improve the current situation. These include increasing access to quality health care services and to education, from early childhood to post-secondary training, resolving housing shortages and food insecurity in the inner city and rural communities, altering our energy system to stop climate change, ending the disproportionate incarceration of Indigenous people, and using a range of economic tools to ensure that everyone can obtain the income we need for healthy lives.

These are broad strokes, and though I have pointed out some examples, they are intentionally short on specifics. The biggest impact will not come from any of my suggestions, but will lie in the realm of democratic reform. If systems are introduced that allow people to become more deeply involved in the process of decision making, they will demand a different approach. They will insist on decisions that improve the health of their families and communities.

This will not happen by accident. If people want a healthy society, they must identify that as their goal and take the necessary steps to make it happen. This means connecting with those who are engaged in civil society and social movements. It means jumping off from the starting point of this book to deeper learning and understanding. It means joining – or forming! – a political party and advocating from within it for greater accountability and democracy. It also means undertaking the difficult task of talking to those with whom we don't agree, of raising the uncomfortable issues of poverty and inequality, and seeking common ground to address them. The idea of a healthy society, particularly one with greater equality, will certainly run up against many detractors. People will find all kinds of reasons why change is not possible, why we must only react to the economically inevitable, why citizens can't be trusted to make wise decisions, why we're stuck.

We're not stuck. There is a lot that can be done, and successful examples abound. First, we need to recognize that we are all in this together. By seeing ourselves as part of a shared project, as working toward a common goal of health, we can create the environment for a new, positive politics. We can establish a functioning means of engaging our challenges and measuring our success in meeting them. This can enable us to improve our meaningful outcomes, to live safer, longer, and happier lives, to enjoy life in a truly healthy society. It can enable us to build our future, together.

NOTES

Preface

1 Quoted in Adrienne Clarkson, *Norman Bethune* (Toronto: Penguin Group, 2009).
2 Michael Marmot, Jessica Allen, and Peter Goldblatt, "A Social Movement, Based on Evidence, to Reduce Inequalities in Health," *Social Science and Medicine* 71, 7 (2010): 1254–58.

Chapter 1: A Healthy Society

1 Commission on Social Determinants of Health, *Closing the Gap in a Generation: Health Equity through Action on the Social Determinants of Health. Final Report of the Commission on Social Determinants of Health* (Geneva: World Health Organization, 2008), http://www.who.int/social_determinants/final_report/csdh_finalreport_2008.pdf.
2 Joseph Lehman, "A Brief Explanation of the Overton Window," Mackinac Center for Public Policy, https://www.mackinac.org/overtonwindow.
3 Frank Newport, "A Tale of Two Supreme Court Decisions" (blog), Gallup, July 2, 2015, http://www.gallup.com/opinion/polling-matters/183908/tale-two-supreme-court-decisions.aspx.
4 George Lakoff, *The All New Don't Think of an Elephant!* (White River Junction, VT: Chelsea Green, 2014), xiv.
5 "Canadians Worried Sick about Health Care," Ekos Politics, October 15, 2015, http://www.ekospolitics.com/index.php/2015/10/canadians-worried-sick-about-health-care.
6 S. Nettleton, "Surveillance, Health Promotion and the Formation of a Risk Identity," in *Debates and Dilemmas in Promoting Health*, ed. M. Sidell et al. (London: Open University Press, 1997), 314–24.

7 Canadian Institute for Health Information, *Improving the Health of Young Canadians: Canadian Population Health Initiative* (Ottawa: Canadian Institute for Health Information, 2005).

8 Dennis Raphael, *Social Determinants of Health: Canadian Perspectives*, 3rd ed. (Toronto: Canadian Scholars' Press, 2016).

9 M. Lemstra, C. Neudorf, and J. Opondo, "Health Disparity by Neighbourhood Income," *Canadian Journal of Public Health* 97, 6 (2006): 435–39.

10 Lemstra, Neudorf, and Opondo, "Health Disparity."

11 Mary Agnes Welch, "Diagnosing Poverty: New Stats Show People in North End Die 16 Years Earlier," *Winnipeg Free Press*, June 6, 2015, https://www.winnipegfreepress.com/local/diagnosing-poverty-306360481.html.

12 "Great Divide of Extremes and Disparity," *Hamilton Spectator*, August 25, 2010, https://www.thespec.com/news-story/2168238-great-divide-of-extremes-and-disparity/.

13 Cory Neudorf et al., "Changes in Social Inequalities in Health over Time in Saskatchewan," 2016, http://saskatchewanequitystudy.com/ses_report_final/.

14 World Health Organization, "Constitution of the World Health Organization: Principles," 1948, http://www.who.int/about/mission/en/l.

15 Richard Wilkinson and Kate Pickett, *The Spirit Level: Why More Equal Societies Almost Always Do Better* (London: Allen Lane, 2009).

16 Editor's Choice, "The Big Idea," *British Medical Journal* 312, 7037 (April 20, 1996), https://doi.org/10.1136/bmj.312.7037.0.

17 Commission on Social Determinants of Health, *Closing the Gap in a Generation*.

Chapter 2: Medicine on a Larger Scale

1 Rudolf Virchow, *Collected Essays on Public Health and Epidemiology* (Canton, MA: Science History, 1985), 33. Originally published 1879.

2 Quoted in Robert F. Woollard, "Caring for a Common Future: Medical Schools' Social Accountability," *Medical Education* 40, 4 (2006): 301, https://doi.org/10.1111/j.1365-2929.2006.02416.x.

3 United Nations, "Universal Declaration of Human Rights," 1948, art. 25(1), http://www.un.org/en/universal-declaration-human-rights/index.html.

4 Sara Gorman, "Inequality, Stress, and Health: The Whitehall Studies," *The Pump Handle*, October 3, 2012, http://scienceblogs.com/thepumphandle/2012/10/03/inequality-stress-and-health-the-whitehall-studies/.

5 Moira A. Stewart et al., *Patient-Centered Medicine: Transforming the Clinical Method* (Thousand Oaks, CA: Sage, 1995).

6 Beth Huntington and Nettie Kuhn, "Communication Gaffes: A Root Cause of Malpractice Claims," *Baylor University Medical Centre Proceedings* 16, 2 (2003): 157–61, https://www.ncbi.nlm.nih.gov/pmc/articles/PMC1201002/.

7 Charles Boelen and Jeffrey E. Heck, *Defining and Measuring Social Accountability of Medical Schools* (Geneva: World Health Organization, 1995).

8   Gordon Guyatt et al., "Evidence-Based Medicine: A New Approach to Teaching the Practice of Medicine," *Journal of the American Medical Association* 268, 17 (1992): 2420–25.

9   RxFiles, http://www.rxfiles.ca.

10   Mark Lemstra and Cory Neudorf, *Health Disparity in Saskatoon: Analysis to Intervention* (Saskatoon: Saskatoon Health Region, 2008).

11   Quoted in Paul Farmer, *Infections and Inequalities: The Modern Plagues* (Berkeley and Los Angeles: University of California Press), 1.

12   Commission on Social Determinants of Health, *Closing the Gap in a Generation: Health Equity through Action on Social Determinants of Health. Final Report of the Commission on the Social Determinants of Health* (Geneva: World Health Organization, 2008), 10, http://www.who.int/social_determinants/final_report/csdh_finalreport_2008.pdf.

13   Eeva Ollila, Fran Baum, and Sebastián Peña, "Introduction to Health in All Policies and the Analytical Framework of the Book," in *Health in All Policies: Seizing Opportunities, Implementing Policies*, ed. Kimmo Leppo et al. (Helsinki: Ministry of Social Affairs and Health, 2013), 3, http://www.euro.who.int/__data/assets/pdf_file/0007/188809/Health-in-All-Policies-final.pdf?ua=1.

14   Louise St-Pierre, *Governance Tools and Framework for Health in All Policies* (The Hague: National Collaborating Centre for Healthy Public Policy, 2009).

15   St-Pierre, *Governance Tools*.

16   "Health Equity Action Lens," Upstream, 2013, http://www.thinkupstream.net/heal1.

Chapter 3: The Extra Mile

1   Ryan Meili, "The Extra Mile," *Canadian Family Physician* 53, 2 (2007): 303–4.

2   Jason R. Frank, Linda Snell, and Jonathan Sherbino, eds., "CanMEDS 2015 Physician Competency Framework," Ottawa, Royal College of Physicians and Surgeons of Canada, 2015, http://www.royalcollege.ca/rcsite/documents/canmeds/canmeds-full-framework-e.pdf.

3   Dom Helder Camara, *Essential Writings* (Maryknoll, NY: Orbis, 2009).

4   "Health and Wealth: Prescribing Money to Treat Low-Income Patients," *The Current*, CBC Radio, November 27, 2013, http://www.cbc.ca/radio/thecurrent/nov-27-2013-1.2909046/health-wealth-prescribing-money-to-treat-low-income-patients-1.2909053.

5   Interview with Gary Bloch, March 2016, conducted by Emily Sullivan.

6   "Poverty: A Clinical Tool for Primary Care Providers," College of Family Physicians of Canada, http://www.cfpc.ca/Poverty_Tools/.

7   "Poverty: A Clinical Tool."

8   "Poverty: A Clinical Tool."

9   Laura McGovern, George Miller, and Paul Hughes-Cromwick, "The Relative Contribution of Multiple Determinants to Health Outcomes," *Health Affairs: Health Policy Brief*, August 21, 2014, http://healthaffairs.org/healthpolicybriefs/brief_pdfs/healthpolicybrief_123.pdf.

10 Sandy Buchman et al., "Practicing Social Accountability: From Theory to Action," *Canadian Family Physician* 62, 1 (2016): 15–18; Ritika Goel et al., "Social Accountability at the Micro Level: One Patient at a Time," *Canadian Family Physician* 62, 4 (2016): 287–90; Robert Woollard et al., "Social Accountability at the Meso Level: Into the Community," *Canadian Family Physician* 62, 7 (2016): 538–40; Ryan Meili et al., "Social Accountability at the Macro Level: Framing the Big Picture," *Canadian Family Physician* 62, 10 (2016): 785–88.

11 Rishi Manchanda, *The Upstream Doctors: Medical Innovators Track Sickness to Its Source* (New York: TED Books, 2013).

12 Bruce Morgan, "Our Ailing Patient," *Tufts Now,* October 14, 2014, http://now. tufts.edu/articles/our-ailing-patient.

13 Manchanda, *Upstream Doctors,* 147.

14 Personal email correspondence between Aidan Halligan and Ryan Meili, 2015.

15 Nicholas Keung, "Refugee Kids' Hospital Admissions Doubled after Ottawa's Health Cuts," *Toronto Star,* May 15, 2014, https://www.thestar.com/news/ investigations/2014/05/15/refugee_kids_hospital_admissions_doubled_after_ ottawas_health_cuts.html.

16 Jonathan Fowlie, "Illegal Billing Identified at Private Vancouver Clinics," *Vancouver Sun,* July 18, 2012, http://www.vancouversun.com/health/Illegal+ billing+identified+private+Vancouver+clinics/6953468/story.html.

17 Michael Marmot, Jessica Allen, and Peter Goldblatt, "A Social Movement, Based on Evidence, to Reduce Inequalities in Health," *Social Science and Medicine* 71, 7 (2010): 1254–58.

18 Upstream, http://www.thinkupstream.net.

19 F. Baum et al., "Social Vaccines to Resist and Change Unhealthy Social and Economic Structures: A Useful Metaphor for Health Promotion," *Health Promotion International* 24, 4 (2009): 428–33.

20 Quoted in Robert F. Woollard, "Caring for a Common Future: Medical Schools' Social Accountability," *Medical Education* 40, 4 (2006): 301, https:// doi.org/10.1111/j.1365-2929.2006.02416.x.

Chapter 4: Growth and Development

1 Juha Mikkonen and Dennis Raphael, "Social Determinants of Health: The Canadian Facts," Toronto, York University School of Health Policy and Management, 2010, 23, http://www.thecanadianfacts.org/the_canadian_ facts.pdf.

2 Dennis Raphael, *Social Determinants of Health: Canadian Perspectives,* 3rd ed. (Toronto: Canadian Scholars' Press, 2016), 9.

3 Robert F. Kennedy, "Remarks at the University of Kansas, March 18, 1968," John F. Kennedy Presidential Library and Museum, https://www.jfklibrary. org/Research/Research-Aids/Ready-Reference/RFK-Speeches/Remarks-of -Robert-F-Kennedy-at-the-University-of-Kansas-March-18-1968.aspx.

4 Joseph Heath, *Filthy Lucre: Economics for People Who Hate Capitalism* (Toronto: Harper Collins, 2009).

5   GPI Atlantic, "The Genuine Progress Index: A Better Set of Tools," September
    14, 2007, http://www.gpiatlantic.org/gpi.htm.
6   Canadian Index of Wellbeing, *How Are Ontarians Really Doing? A Provincial
    Report on Ontario Wellbeing*, Waterloo, ON, University of Waterloo, April
    2014, https://uwaterloo.ca/canadian-index-wellbeing/sites/ca.canadian-index
    -wellbeing/files/uploads/files/ontarioreport-accessible_o.pdf.
7   Canadian Index of Wellbeing, *How are Canadians Really Doing? The 2016
    CIW National Report*, Waterloo, ON, University of Waterloo, Faculty of Applied
    Health Sciences, https://uwaterloo.ca/canadian-index-wellbeing/sites/ca.
    canadian-index-wellbeing/files/uploads/files/co11676-nationalreport-ciw_
    final-s_o.pdf.
8   M. Lemstra, C. Neudorf, and J. Opondo, "Health Disparity by Neighbourhood
    Income," *Canadian Journal of Public Health* 97, 6 (2006): 435–39.
9   Broadbent Institute, "The Wealth Gap: Perceptions and Misconceptions
    in Canada," December 2014, https://d3n8a8pro7vhmx.cloudfront.net/
    broadbent/pages/31/attachments/original/1430002077/The_Wealth_Gap.pdf?
    1430002077.
10 Broadbent Institute, "The Wealth Gap."
11 OECD, "Focus on Inequality and Growth," December 2014, https://www.oecd.
    org/els/soc/Focus-Inequality-and-Growth-2014.pdf.
12 Canada Mortgage and Housing Corporation, "Housing Market Indicators,
    Canada, Provinces, and Metropolitan Areas, 1990–2016," https://www.cmhc
    -schl.gc.ca/en/hoficlincl/homain/stda/data/data_001.cfm.
13 Canadian Housing Observer, "Housing Market Indicators."
14 Paul Gingrich, "Boom and Bust: The Growing Income Gap in Saskatchewan,"
    Regina, Canadian Centre for Policy Alternatives, September 2009, https://
    www.policyalternatives.ca/publications/reports/boom-and-bust.
15 Gingrich, "Boom and Bust."
16 Cory Neudorf et al., "Changes in Social Inequalities in Health over Time
    in Saskatchewan," 2016, http://saskatchewanequitystudy.com/ses_report
    _final/.
17 Eric W. Kierans, "Globalism and the Nation-State," in *The Lost Massey Lectures:
    Recovered Classics from Five Great Thinkers* (Toronto: House of Anansi Press,
    2007), 258.
18 J. Székács Jacobi, *Selected Writings by Paracelsus* (Princeton: Bollingen Founda-
    tion Collection, 1995), 63.
19 Daniel Munro, "Healthy People, Healthy Performance, Healthy Profits: The
    Case for Business Action on the Socio-economic Determinants of Health,"
    Ottawa, Conference Board of Canada, December 2008, http://www.
    conferenceboard.ca/Libraries/NETWORK_PUBLIC/dec2008_report_
    healthypeople.sflb.
20 Harry J. Holzer et al., "The Economic Costs of Poverty in the United States:
    Subsequent Effects of Children Growing Up Poor," Institute for Research on
    Poverty Discussion Paper 1327-07, April 2007, https://www.irp.wisc.edu/
    publications/dps/pdfs/dp132707.pdf.

21 Nathan Laurie, "The Cost of Poverty: An Analysis of the Economic Cost of Poverty in Ontario," Toronto, Ontario Association of Food Banks, November 2008, https://www.oafb.ca/assets/pdfs/CostofPoverty.pdf.

22 Commission on Social Determinants of Health, *Closing the Gap in a Generation: Health Equity through Action on the Social Determinants of Health. Final Report of the Commission on Social Determinants of Health* (Geneva: World Health Organization, 2008), http://www.who.int/social_determinants/final_report/csdh_finalreport_2008.pdf.

23 Sarath Peiris, "Saskatchewan's 'Austerity Budget' Comes Too Late," *CBC News,* March 22, 2017, http://www.cbc.ca/news/canada/saskatchewan/saskatchewan-s-austerity-budget-comes-too-late-1.4036468.

24 Government of Canada, Department of Finance, "Annex 1: Job Impact of the Economic Action Plan to Date," 2010, http://www.budget.gc.ca/2010/plan/anx1-eng.html.

25 Nick Falvo, "Saskatchewan's Budget Is Robin Hood in Reverse," *Regina Leader-Post,* April 22, 2017, http://leaderpost.com/opinion/columnists/saskatchewans-budget-is-robin-hood-in-reverse.

26 Kenneth Boulding, *Energy Reorganization Act of 1973: Hearings,* Ninety-third Congress, first session, 1973 (Washington, DC: US Government Printing Office, 1973).

27 During an interview with the *Toronto Globe and Mail,* Harper said, "You know, there's two schools in economics on this, one is that there are some good taxes and the other is that no taxes are good taxes. I'm in the latter category. I don't believe any taxes are good taxes." "What Harper Told the Globe," *Toronto Globe and Mail,* July 10, 2009, https://beta.theglobeandmail.com/news/politics/what-harper-told-the-globe/article4278789/?ref=http://www.theglobeandmail.com&.

28 Hugh Mackenzie and Richard Shillington, "Canada's Quiet Bargain: The Benefits of Public Spending," Ottawa, Canadian Centre for Policy Alternatives, April 2009, https://www.policyalternatives.ca/publications/reports/canadas-quiet-bargain.

29 Jonathan D. Ostry, Andrew Berg, and Charalambos G. Tsangarides, "Redistribution, Inequality, and Growth," IMF Staff Discussion Note, International Monetary Fund, February 2014, http://www.imf.org/external/pubs/ft/sdn/2014/sdn1402.pdf.

30 Mariana Mazzucato, *The Entrepreneurial State: Debunking Public vs. Private Sector Myths* (New York: Anthem Press, 2013).

31 "Lorne Calvert Wraps Up Career in Legislature," *CBC News,* May 14, 2009, http://www.cbc.ca/news/canada/saskatchewan/story/2009/05/14/calvert-final-day.html.

Chapter 5: The Search for a Cure to Poverty

1 Dennis Raphael and Toba Bryant, "The Health Effects of Income Inequality: A Jet with 110 Canadians Falling Out of the Sky Each Day, Every Day, 365 Days a Year," *Upstream,* November 25, 2014.

2   Raphael and Bryant, "The Health Effects of Income Inequality."

3   "Just the Facts," Canada without Poverty, 2015, http://www.cwp-csp.ca/poverty/ just-the-facts/; Nathan Laurie, "The Cost of Poverty: An Analysis of the Economic Cost of Poverty in Ontario," Toronto, Ontario Association of Food Banks, November 2008, https://www.oafb.ca/assets/pdfs/CostofPoverty.pdf.

4   K. Hammond et al., "Increasing Burden of HIV/AIDS on Hospitals in Sas-katoon, Saskatchewan, Canada" (poster presented at Infectious Diseases Society of America annual meeting, Boston, 2011).

5   Perri Klass, "Poverty as a Childhood Disease," Well (blog), *New York Times*, May 13, 2013, https://well.blogs.nytimes.com/2013/05/13/poverty-as-a -childhood-disease/?mcubz=3.

6   Ryan Meili, "Public Health Is Getting Political," *Huffington Post* (blog), November 25, 2014, http://www.huffingtonpost.ca/ryan-meili/public-health -policy-canada_b_6209524.html.

7   Canadian Medical Association, "Physicians and Health Equity: Opportunities in Practice," Ottawa, Canadian Medical Association, 2013, https://www.cma. ca/Assets/assets-library/document/en/advocacy/Health-Equity-Opportunities -in-Practice-Final-e.pdf.

8   Charles Plante and Keisha Sharp, *Poverty Costs Saskatchewan: A New Approach to Prosperity for All* (Saskatoon: Poverty Costs, 2014).

9   Laurie, "The Cost of Poverty."

10 Advisory Group on Poverty Reduction, "Recommendations for a Provincial Poverty Reduction Strategy," 2015, https://www.saskatchewan.ca/~/media/ news%20release%20backgrounders/2015/aug/advisory%20group%20on %20poverty%20reduction%20report.pdf.

11 Evelyn L. Forget, "The Town with No Poverty: The Health Effects of a Can-adian Guaranteed Annual Income Field Experiment," *Canadian Public Policy* 37, 3 (2011): 283–305.

12 Forget, "The Town with No Poverty."

13 Canadian Institute for Health Information, "National Health Expenditure Trends, 1975 to 2016," 2016, https://www.cihi.ca/sites/default/files/document/ nhex-trends-narrative-report_2016_en.pdf.

14 David Shum, "Ontario Basic Income Pilot Project to Be Tested in Hamilton, Lindsay, Thunder Bay," *Global News*, April 24, 2017, http://globalnews.ca/ news/3399143/ontario-basic-income-pilot-project/.

15 Evelyn L. Forget, "Do We Still Need a Basic Income Guarantee in Canada?" Basic Income Guarantee Series, Research Paper 22, Thunder Bay, ON, Northern Policy Institute, 2017, http://www.northernpolicy.ca/upload/ documents/publications/research-reports/paper-forget-big-en-17.05.29.pdf.

16 A. Reeves et al., "Does Investment in the Health Sector Promote or Inhibit Economic Growth?" *Globalization and Health* 9, 43 (2013): 3.

17 Ryan Meili and James Hughes, "Accounting Rules Need to Allow the Amortization of Social Investments," *Toronto Globe and Mail*, August 12, 2016, https://www.theglobeandmail.com/report-on-business/rob-commentary/ accounting-rules-need-to-allow-the-amortization-of-social-investments/ article31378871/.

18 Armine Yalnizyan, "Why a $15 Minimum Wage Is Good for Business," *Maclean's,* June 2, 2017, http://www.macleans.ca/economy/economicanalysis/why-a-15-minimum-wage-is-good-for-business/.

19 George Wehby, Dhaval Dave, and Robert Kaestner, "Effects of the Minimum Wage on Infant Health" (working paper, National Bureau of Economic Research, Cambridge, MA, 2016), http://www.nber.org/papers/w22373.pdf.

20 Living Wage Saskatoon, "About," http://www.livingwageyxe.ca/about.

Chapter 6: Out of House and Home

1   Stephen Gaetz, Tanya Gulliver, and Tim Richter, "The State of Homelessness in Canada, 2014," Homeless Hub Paper 5, Toronto, Homeless Hub, 2014, http://homelesshub.ca/sites/default/files/SOHC2014.pdf.

2   J. David Hulchanski, *Housing Policy for Tomorrow's Cities* (Ottawa: Canadian Policy Research Networks, 2002).

3   Federation of Canadian Municipalities, "Sustaining the Momentum: Recommendations for a National Action Plan on Housing and Homelessness," January 2008, https://www.fcm.ca/Documents/reports/Sustaining_the_Momentum_Recommendations_for_a_National_Action_Plan_on_Housing_and_Homelessness_EN.pdf.

4   Government of Canada, "Highlights of the National Shelter Study, 2005–2014," 2016, https://www.canada.ca/en/employment-social-development/programs/communities/homelessness/reports-shelter-2014.html.

5   Government of Canada, "Highlights of the National Shelter Study."

6   "Number of Homeless Children in Saskatoon Up," *CBC News,* August 19, 2015, http://www.cbc.ca/news/canada/saskatoon/number-of-homeless-children-in-saskatoon-up-1.3196853.

7   Gaetz, Gulliver, and Richter, "The State of Homelessness."

8   Erika Khandor and Kate Mason, "The Street Health Report 2007," Toronto, Wellesley Institute, 2007, http://www.wellesleyinstitute.com/wp-content/uploads/2007/09/Street-Health-Report-2007.pdf.

9   Stephanie Levitz, "Canadian Homelessness: $46 a Person Would Help, Report Says," *CBC News,* October 29, 2014, http://www.cbc.ca/news/canada/canadian-homelessness-46-a-person-would-help-report-says-1.2816663.

10 Canadian Press, "Homeless People's Life Expectancy Half of Average in B.C.," *CBC News,* November 6, 2014, http://www.cbc.ca/news/canada/british-columbia/homeless-people-s-life-expectancy-half-of-average-in-b-c-1.2826335.

11 Gaetz, Gulliver, and Richter, "The State of Homelessness."

12 Christina Haddad, "Have Your Say in Shaping the Future of Housing in Canada," *Ottawa Sun,* August 5, 2016, http://www.ottawasun.com/2016/08/05/have-your-say-in-shaping-the-future-of-housing-in-canada.

13 Jordan Press, "Expectations High for Proposed National Housing Strategy, CMHC Says," *Vancouver Metro News,* September 6, 2016, http://www.metronews.ca/news/canada/2016/09/06/expectations-high-for-proposed-national-housing-strategy-cmhc-says.html.

14 Stephen Gaetz, Fiona Scott, and Tanya Gulliver, eds., "Housing First in Canada: Supporting Communities to End Homelessness," Toronto, Canadian Homelessness Research Network Press, 2013, http://www.homelesshub.ca/sites/default/files/HousingFirstInCanada.pdf.

15 Kendall Latimer, "'It Absolutely Works': Housing First Marks 1 Year in Regina," *CBC News,* July 18, 2017, http://www.cbc.ca/news/canada/saskatchewan/housing-first-regina-homelessness-one-year-1.4210744.

16 Sarah Lawrynuik, "Medicine Hat Maintaining Homeless-Free Status 2 Years On," *CBC News,* January 26, 2017, http://www.cbc.ca/news/canada/calgary/medicine-hat-homeless-free-update-1.3949030.

17 "Medicine Hat Becomes the First Canadian City to Eliminate Homelessness," *As It Happens,* CBC Radio, May 14, 2015, http://www.cbc.ca/radio/asithappens/as-it-happens-thursday-edition-1.3074402/medicine-hat-becomes-the-first-city-in-canada-to-eliminate-homelessness-1.3074742.

18 Valerie Tarasuk, Andy Mitchell, and Naomi Dachner, "Household Food Insecurity in Canada, 2014," Toronto, Research to Identify Policy Options to Reduce Food Insecurity, 2014, http://proof.utoronto.ca/wp-content/uploads/2016/04/Household-Food-Insecurity-in-Canada-2014.pdf.

19 Urshila Sriram and Valerie Tarasuk, "Economic Predictors of Household Food Insecurity in Canadian Metropolitan Areas," *Journal of Hunger and Environmental Nutrition* 11, 1 (2016): 1–13, https://doi.org/10.1080/19320248.2015.1045670.

20 Tarasuk, Mitchell, and Dachner, "Household Food Insecurity."

21 Tarasuk, Mitchell, and Dachner, "Household Food Insecurity."

22 Valerie Tarasuk et al., "Association between Household Food Insecurity and Annual Health Care Costs," *Canadian Medical Association Journal* 187, 14 (2015): E429–36.

23 Val Tarasuk, "The Full Story of Food (In)security" (paper presented at Closing the Gap Conference, Ottawa, April 30, 2016), https://www.youtube.com/watch?v=CnOwZS2D0GY.

24 Joel Novek, "CED Food Initiatives in Inner City Saskatoon and Winnipeg: Very Much Alive at the Twenty Year Mark," Winnipeg, Canadian Centre for Policy Alternatives, 2009, https://www.policyalternatives.ca/sites/default/files/uploads/publications/reports/docs/CED_Food_Initiatives_111509.pdf.

25 Saskatchewan Food Costing Task Group, "The Cost of Healthy Eating in Saskatchewan," 2015, https://www.dietitians.ca/Downloads/Public/2015-The-Cost-of-Healthy-Eating-in-Saskatchewan.aspx.

Chapter 7: The Warming World

1 Kate Raworth, *Doughnut Economics: Seven Ways to Think Like a 21st Century Economist* (White River Junction, VT: Chelsea Green, 2016).

2 Canadian Public Health Association, "Global Change and Public Health: Addressing the Ecological Determinants of Health," Canadian Public Health Association Discussion Paper, May 2015, https://www.cpha.ca/sites/default/files/assets/policy/edh-discussion_e.pdf.

3 "Climate Change and Human Health," World Health Organization, 2015, http://www.who.int/globalchange/global-campaign/cop21/en/.

4 Inter-American Commission on Human Rights, *Report on the Situation of Human Rights in Brazil, 1997,* http://www.cidh.org/countryrep/brazil-eng/index%20-%20brazil.htm.

5 Conference Board of Canada, "How Canada Performs: Greenhouse Gas (GHG) Emissions," April 2016, http://www.conferenceboard.ca/hcp/provincial/environment/ghg-emissions.aspx.

6 N. Watts et al., "Health and Climate Change: Policy Responses to Protect Public Health," *Lancet* 386, 10006 (2015): 1905.

7 "Resolutions Adopted (Confirmed)," 148th annual meeting of the Canadian Medical Association, 2015, https://www.cma.ca/Assets/assets-library/document/en/about-us/gc2015/resolutions-passed-at-gc_final_english.pdf.

8 Government of Canada, "Pricing Carbon Pollution in Canada: How It Will Work," 2016, https://www.canada.ca/en/environment-climate-change/news/2017/05/pricing_carbon_pollutionincanadahowitwillwork.html.

9 Canadian Labour Congress, "One Million Climate Jobs: A Challenge for Canada," 2016, http://greeneconomynet.ca/wp-content/uploads/sites/43/2014/07/OneMilClimateJobs-Backgrounder-2016-11-01-EN.pdf.

10 Government of Alberta, "Carbon Levy and Rebates," 2016, https://www.alberta.ca/climate-carbon-pricing.aspx.

11 Aleszu Bajak, "Reframing Climate Change as a Public Health Threat," Undark.org, September 16, 2016, https://undark.org/2016/09/16/framing-climate-change-as-a-public-health-threat/.

Chapter 8: The Equality of Mercy

1 "Ex-Posse Kingpin Turns Life Around," *Saskatoon StarPhoenix,* August 28, 2010.

2 Ross Gordon Green and Kearney Healy, *Tough on Kids: Rethinking Approaches to Youth Justice* (Saskatoon: Purich Publishing, 2003).

3 "Aboriginal People Over-Represented in Saskatchewan's Prisons," Statistics Canada, *Canada Year Book,* 2006, http://www.statcan.gc.ca/pub/11-402-x/2006/2693/ceb2693_002-eng.htm.

4 "Canada's Prison Farm System Being Phased Out," *CBC News,* February 25, 2009, www.cbc.ca/news/canada/ottawa/story/2009/02/25/prison-farms.html.

5 Don Healy, "Saskatchewan Premier Tells 115 Inmates Refusing to Eat How to Avoid Prison Food – Don't Go to Jail," *National Post,* January 7, 2016, http://nationalpost.com/news/canada/saskatchewan-premier-tells-115-inmates-refusing-to-eat-how-to-avoid-prison-food-dont-go-to-jail/wcm/2c0457dc-ee55-444a-9658-2696eab4aee3.

6 Institute for Criminal Policy Research, "United States of America," *World Prison Brief,* 2014, http://www.prisonstudies.org/country/united-states-america.

7 David Cayley, *The Expanding Prison: The Crisis in Crime and Punishment and the Search for Alternatives* (Toronto: House of Anansi Press, 1998), 67.

8   Richard Wilkinson and Kate Pickett, *The Spirit Level: Why More Equal Societies Almost Always Do Better* (London: Allen Lane, 2009), 149.

9   Donna Calverley, "Adult Correctional Services in Canada 2008/2009," *Juristat* 30, 3 (Fall 2010), http://www.statcan.gc.ca/pub/85-002-x/2010003/article/11353-eng.pdf.

10 Calverley, "Adult Correctional Services."

11 Paula Smith, Claire Goggin, and Paul Gendreau, "The Effects of Prison Sentences and Intermediate Sanctions on Recidivism: General Effects and Individual Differences," User Report 2002-01, Solicitor General Canada, 2002, https://www.publicsafety.gc.ca/cnt/rsrcs/pblctns/ffcts-prsn-sntncs/ffcts-prsn-sntncs-eng.pdf.

12 Institute for Criminal Policy Research, *World Prison Brief.*

13 ChartsBin, "Current Worldwide Homicide/Murder Rate," http://chartsbin.com/view/1454.

14 Green and Healy, *Tough on Kids.*

15 Andréa Ledding, "Getting Tough on Crime the Wrong Focus: Weighill," *Prairie Messenger*, April 14, 2010.

16 Author conversation with Kearney Healy, Saskatoon legal aid lawyer and co-author of *Tough on Kids*, May 2011.

17 Ledding, "Getting Tough on Crime."

18 Ledding, "Getting Tough on Crime."

19 Ledding, "Getting Tough on Crime."

20 Shawn Atleo, "Point of View: There Is an Election On, Isn't It Time We Talked?" *CBC News*, April 13, 2011, http://www.cbc.ca/news/canada/story/2011/04/13/cv-election-atleo-oped.html.

21 Chad Nilson, *Risk-Driven Collaborative Intervention: A Preliminary Impact Assessment of Community Mobilization Prince Albert's Hub Model* (Saskatoon: Centre for Forensic Behavioural Science and Justice Studies, University of Saskatchewan, 2014), https://www.usask.ca/cfbsjs/research/pdf/research_reports/RiskDrivenCollaborativeIntervention.pdf.

22 "Who We Are: The Scottish Influence," Prince Albert Community Mobilization, 2015, http://www.mobilizepa.ca/who-we-are/the-scottish-influence.

23 Emma Young, "Iceland Knows How to Stop Teen Substance Abuse but the World Isn't Listening," Mosaic Science, January 2017, https://mosaicscience.com/story/iceland-prevent-teen-substance-abuse.

24 Ledding, "Getting Tough on Crime."

Chapter 9: Learning to Live

1   *Life and Works of Horace Mann*, ed. Mary Mann (Boston: Walker, Fuller, 1868), 669.

2   First Nations Child and Family Caring Society of Canada, "Shannen's Dream," https://fncaringsociety.com/shannens-dream.

3   Charlie Angus, "What If They Declared an Emergency and No One Came?" *Huffington Post* (blog), November 21, 2011, http://www.huffingtonpost.ca/charlie-angus/attawapiskat-emergency_b_1104370.html.

4   "Fact Sheet: First Nations Education Funding," Assembly of First Nations, 2011, http://www.afn.ca/uploads/files/education/2._k-12_first_nations_education_funding_fact_sheet,_afn_2011.pdf.

5   "Undergraduate Tuition Fees for Full Time Canadian Students, by Discipline, by Province (Saskatchewan)," Statistics Canada, 2016, http://www.statcan.gc.ca/tables-tableaux/sum-som/l01/cst01/educ50i-eng.htm.

6   Marc Frenette, "Postsecondary Enrolment by Parental Income: Recent National and Provincial Trends," Statistics Canada, April 10, 2017, http://www.statcan.gc.ca/pub/11-626-x/11-626-x2017070-eng.htm.

7   Nick Martin, "U of M Looking to Make Changes to Medical School Admissions in 2016," *Winnipeg Free Press*, May 12, 2015, https://www.winnipegfreepress.com/local/U-of-M-looking-to-make-changes-to-medical-school-admission-in-2016-303522391.html.

8   Roger Martin, "Who Killed Canada's Education Advantage," *Walrus Magazine*, November 2009.

9   C.B. Koester, ed., *The Measure of the Man: Selected Speeches of Woodrow Stanley Lloyd* (Winnipeg: Western Producer Prairie Books, 1976).

10 Saskatchewan Human Rights Commission, "Citizenship Education," http://saskatchewanhumanrights.ca/learn/citizenship-education.

11 Joel Westheimer, "No Child Left Thinking: Democracy at Risk in Canadian Schools" (videotaped presentation to the Department of Education, University of Regina, January 2010), http://vimeo.com/9054678.

12 Juha Mikkonen and Dennis Raphael, "Social Determinants of Health: The Canadian Facts," Toronto, York University School of Health Policy and Management, 2010, 23, http://www.thecanadianfacts.org/the_canadian_facts.pdf.

13 Paul Kershaw, "Does Canada Work for All Generations?" Human Early Learning Partnership, University of British Columbia, Fall 2011, http://earlylearning.ubc.ca/media/publications/Family%20Policy%20Reports%20and%20Resources/does_canada_work_for_all_generations_national_summary.pdf.

14 Jane Beach et al., *Early Childhood Education and Care in Canada 2008*, 8th ed., Childcare Resource and Research Unit, 2009, http://www.childcarecanada.org/ECEC2008/index.html.

15 Laurie Monsebraaten, "Quebec's Child-Care Scheme Pays for Itself, Economist," *Toronto Star*, June 22, 2011, https://www.thestar.com/life/parent/2011/06/22/quebecs_childcare_scheme_pays_for_itself_economist.html.

16 Alan C. O'Connor et al., "Economic Impact Analysis of the University of Saskatchewan: Final Report," September 2015, https://www.usask.ca/ipa/documents/resource-allocation/RTI-UofS__12-30_no_appendix_optimized.pdf.

17 M. Coelli, "Tuition Fees and Equality of Enrollment," *Canadian Journal of Economics* 42, 3 (2009): 1078.

18 Christine Neill, "What You Don't Know Can't Help You: Lessons of Behavioural Economics for Tax-Based Student Aid," C.D. Howe Institute Commentary 393, November 2013, https://www.cdhowe.org/sites/default/files/attachments/research_papers/mixed/Commentary_393_0.pdf.

1   Jeff Turnbull, "Building a Stronger, Sustainable Medicare for Canadians" (AFMC-AFS Wendell MacLeod Memorial Lecture, Toronto, May 15, 2011).

2   Laura McGovern, George Miller, and Paul Hughes-Cromwick, "The Relative Contribution of Multiple Determinants to Health Outcomes," *Health Affairs: Health Policy Brief,* August 21, 2014, http://healthaffairs.org/healthpolicybriefs/brief_pdfs/healthpolicybrief_123.pdf.

3   Juha Mikkonen and Dennis Raphael, "Social Determinants of Health: The Canadian Facts," Toronto, York University School of Health Policy and Management, 2010, http://www.thecanadianfacts.org/the_canadian_facts.pdf.

4   Charles Boelen and Jeffrey E. Heck, *Defining and Measuring Social Accountability of Medical Schools* (Geneva: World Health Organization, 1995), 3.

5   Ryan Meili et al., "The CARE Model of Social Accountability: Promoting Cultural Change," *Academic Medicine* 86 (2011): 1114–19.

6   "Health Expenditure as a Share of GDP, 1960-2009, Selected OECD Countries," *Health at a Glance 2011: OECD Indicators,* OECD, 2011, 12, https://www.oecd.org/els/health-systems/49105858.pdf.

7   Commission on the Future of Health Care in Canada, *Building on Values: The Future of Health Care in Canada – Final Report,* xvi, Ottawa, November 2002. http://publications.gc.ca/collections/Collection/CP32-85-2002E.pdf.

8   Commission on the Future of Health Care in Canada, *Building on Values*; Maude Barlow, *Profit Is Not the Cure* (Toronto: McClelland and Stewart, 2001).

9   "Health Spending," OECD Health Data, 2014, https://data.oecd.org/healthres/health-spending.htm.

10 Canadian Institute for Health Information, *Drug Expenditure in Canada, 1985 to 2010* (Ottawa, 2011).

11 Steve Morgan et al., "Estimated Cost of Universal Public Coverage of Prescription Drugs in Canada," *Canadian Medical Association Journal* 187, 7 (April 2015): 491–97.

12 Reed F. Beall, Jason W. Nickerson, and Amir Attaran, "Pan-Canadian Overpricing of Medicines: A 6-Country Study of Cost Control for Generic Medicines," *Open Medicine* 8, 4 (2014): 131.

13 Jane Taber, "National Pharmacare Has Large Support across Canada, Poll Says," *Toronto Globe and Mail,* July 15, 2015, https://www.theglobeandmail.com/news/national/national-pharmacare-has-large-support-across-canada-says-poll/article25509989/.

14 "Prescription Drug Access and Affordability an Issue for Nearly a Quarter of All Canadian Households," Angus Reid Institute, July 15, 2015, http://angusreid.org/prescription-drugs-canada/.

15 Health Council of Canada, "Better Health, Better Care, Better Value for All: Refocusing Health Care Reform in Canada," September 2013.

16 Canadian Institute for Health Information, "National Health Expenditure Trends, 1975 to 2016," 2016, https://www.cihi.ca/sites/default/files/document/nhex-trends-narrative-report_2016_en.pdf.

17 Mark Lemstra and Cory Neudorf, *Health Disparity in Saskatoon: Analysis to Intervention* (Saskatoon: Saskatoon Health Region, 2008).

18 Atul Gawande, "The Hot Spotters: Can We Lower Medical Costs by Giving the Neediest Patients Better Care?" *New Yorker,* January 24, 2011, http://www.newyorker.com/magazine/2011/01/24/the-hot-spotters.

19 Ryan Meili, "How Do We Cool Down Canada's 'Medical Hot Spots'?" *Huffington Post* (blog), January 25, 2014, http://www.huffingtonpost.ca/ryan-meili/canada-healthcare_b_4312263.html.

20 Brian Goldman, "Medical Hotspot: Saskatoon, Saskatchewan," *White Coat Black Art,* CBC Radio, December 1, 2012, http://www.cbc.ca/player/play/2311645308.

Chapter 11: Less Politics, More Democracy

1 Commission on Social Determinants of Health, *Closing the Gap in a Generation: Health Equity through Action on the Social Determinants of Health. Final Report of the Commission on Social Determinants of Health* (Geneva: World Health Organization, 2008), http://www.who.int/social_determinants/final_report/csdh_finalreport_2008.pdf.

2 Canada, Standing Senate Committee on Social Affairs, Science and Technology, Subcommittee on Population Health, *A Healthy, Productive Canada: A Determinant of Health Approach* (Ottawa: Author, 2009), https://sencanada.ca/content/sen/Committee/402/popu/rep/rephealth1jun09-e.pdf.

3 G. Dickson, "Participatory Action Research: Theory and Practice," in *Community Nursing: Promoting Canadians' Health,* 2nd ed., ed. M. Stewart (Toronto: W.B. Saunders, 2000), 542–63.

4 Cindy Blackstock, "Justice Long Overdue for First Nations," presentation, Upstream Closing the Gap Conference, Ottawa, April 4, 2016.

5 Truth and Reconciliation Commission of Canada, "Calls to Action," Winnipeg, Truth and Reconciliation Commission of Canada, 2015, http://www.trc.ca/websites/trcinstitution/File/2015/Findings/Calls_to_Action_English2.pdf.

6 Quoted in "Quotes about the Truth and Reconciliation Commission Report," *Vancouver Metro,* June 2, 2015, http://www.metronews.ca/news/canada/2015/06/02/words-of-truth-and-reconciliation.html.

7 First Nations Child and Family Caring Society of Canada, "Jordan's Principle," 2014, https://fncaringsociety.com/jordans-principle.

8 First Nations Child and Family Caring Society of Canada, "Jordan's Principle," https://fncaringsociety.com/jordans-principle.

9 Advisory Group on Poverty Reduction, "Recommendations for a Provincial Poverty Reduction Strategy," 2015, https://www.saskatchewan.ca/~/media/news%20release%20backgrounders/2015/aug/advisory%20group%20on%20poverty%20reduction%20report.pdf.

10 Melisa Brittain and Cindy Blackstock, *First Nations Child Poverty: A Literature Review and Analysis,* First Nations Children's Action Research and Education

Service, 2015, https://fncaringsociety.com/sites/default/files/First%20
Nations%20Child%20Poverty%20-%20A%20Literature%20Review%20
and%20Analysis%202015-3.pdf.

11 Truth and Reconciliation Commission of Canada, "Calls to Action."

12 *First Nations Child and Family Caring Society of Canada et al. v. Attorney General of Canada*, 2016 CHRT 2, Canadian Human Rights Tribunal, 2016, http://decisions.chrt-tcdp.gc.ca/chrt-tcdp/decisions/en/item/127700/index.do?r=AAAAAQALMjAxNiBDSFJUIDIB.

13 Marina Jiménez, "Pharma Freebies Sway Med Students," *Toronto Globe and Mail,* May 11, 2009, https://theglobeandmail.com/life/health-and-fitness/pharma-freebies-sway-med-students/article1196164/?ref=http://www.theglobeandmail.com&.

14 David Grande, "Limiting the Influence of Pharmaceutical Industry Gifts on Physicians: Self-Regulation or Government Intervention?" *Journal of General Internal Medicine* 25, 1 (2010): 81.

15 Daniel Tencer, "Canada's Most and Least Trusted Professions: Sorry, CEOs and Politicians," *Huffington Post,* January 20, 2015, http://www.huffingtonpost.ca/2015/01/20/most-least-trusted-professions-canada_n_6510232.html.

16 Progress Alberta, "Brad Wall Took Money from Who?" November 1, 2016, http://www.progressalberta.ca/brad_wall_took_money_from_who.

17 Mainstreet Research, "Political Financing in Saskatchewan," Blog, November 4, 2016, http://www.mainstreetresearch.ca/political-financing/.

18 Charles Smith and Ryan Meili, "Opinion: Saskatchewan's Political Donation Problem Is a Caution for Canada," *Toronto Globe and Mail,* November 4, 2016, https://theglobeandmail.com/opinion/saskatchewans-political-donation-problem-is-a-caution-for-canada/article32690615/?ref=http://www.theglobeandmail.com&.

19 Chris Koentges, "The Campaign in Full Sentences," SwerveCalgary.com, http://themagazineschool.ca/files/2011/TheCampaigninFullSentences.pdf.

Chapter 12: Our Future Together

1 Commission on the Future of Health Care in Canada, *Building on Values: The Future of Health Care in Canada – Final Report,* Ottawa, November 2002, http://publications.gc.ca/collections/Collection/CP32-85-2002E.pdf.

2 Juha Mikkonen and Dennis Raphael, "Social Determinants of Health: The Canadian Facts," Toronto, York University School of Health Policy and Management, 2010, 23, http://www.thecanadianfacts.org/the_canadian_facts.pdf.

3 M. Lemstra, C. Neudorf, and G. Beaudin, "Health Disparity Knowledge and Support for Intervention in Saskatoon," *Canadian Journal of Public Health* 98 (2007): 484–88.

4 Dennis Raphael, "Escaping from the *Phantom Zone:* Social Determinants of Health, Public Health Units and Public Policy in Canada," *Health Promotion International* 24, 2 (2009): 194. In the *Superman* movies, the Phantom Zone is

an other-dimensional prison in which three arch-criminals are permanently incarcerated. It is hurled into the obscurity of deep space.

5 Canadian Medical Association, "Health Care in Canada: What Makes Us Sick?" Town Hall Report, July 2013, https://www.cma.ca/Assets/assets-library/document/fr/advocacy/What-makes-us-sick_en.pdf.

ACKNOWLEDGMENTS

Each patient story in this work is true in concept, but each has also been altered somewhat: the names and physical details have been changed to protect the privacy and confidentiality of all involved. Whenever possible, I discussed the inclusion of the story with the patient. The ability to share in the lives of so many people, in intimate moments of birth and death, illness and cure, sadness and joy, is the greatest privilege of life as a physician. These interactions continue to teach me about life and how to live it, and I'm sincerely grateful to all who have shared their stories, their strengths, and their vulnerabilities with me throughout my training and practice.

While most books show the name of a single author under the title, they are generally the product of many minds. *A Healthy Society* is an extreme example thereof, as I have leaned heavily and repeatedly on the advice and input of friends, family, and colleagues in its preparation. Much of this leaning occurred long before any thought of producing a book. Rather, it was the countless classes, long walks, road trips, phone conversations, recommended readings, and fiery debates in which ideas and opinions were formed, smashed, and reshaped. To thank everyone who was and is a part of that process would be a tome in itself. If you see yourself in the book, be sure that I do too.

As for the textual manifestation of that process, my sincere thanks go to all those who reviewed the work in whole or in part and shared their advice. Thank you to William Albritton, Doris Dick, Erika Dyck, Noah Evanchuk, Max Fineday, Chris Gallaway, Cory Neudorf, David Forbes, Mark Lemstra, Nazeem Muhajarine, Father Les Paquin, Bill Peterson, Peter Prebble, Brendan Pyle, and Jeff and Fleur MacQueen Smith; to my parents, Wally and Lea Meili; and to my oldest and most loyal friend, Paul Rowe. Deserving of special mention is Kearney Healy, one of Canada's finer minds in the pursuit of justice, for his substantial contribution to the ideas presented in the chapter on justice.

In the years between the first and second edition, I wrote op-eds on various topics for publications across Canada as an Evidence Network expert and Broadbent Institute fellow, and in my roles at the University of Saskatchewan and Upstream. Some of these were solo articles, others were co-written. I have used some of the ideas and writing from these articles in this latest edition. When that content came from jointly written pieces, it has been shared with and approved by the original co-authors. My thanks to Monika Dutt, Christine Gibson, Nigel Hewitt, Courtney Howard, James Hughes, Julio Montaner, Danyaal Raza, Tim Richter, and Michael Schwandt for sharing this work with me, as well as my colleagues with the Social Accountability Working Group. Thanks to Emily Sullivan for interviewing Gary Bloch and Andrew Pinto regarding the St. Michael's project and Poverty Assessment Tool.

Going beyond the immediate contributions to the book at hand, I'm inclined to reflect on the development of my thought and practice on how best to work with communities. Looking back, there are some key role models who must be acknowledged. Fathers Don McGillivray and Les Paquin, through their work in northeastern Brazil, demonstrated how to live humbly among the poor and to work boldly for justice. The work of Drs. Gerri and Murray Dickson with communities in rural Mozambique has been an extraordinary example of honest and open partnership in pursuit of healthy development. Dr. William Albritton, dean of the College of Medicine in Saskatoon, has been an incredible support and mentor in the development of my understanding of leadership and social accountability. Physicians who dedicate their lives to their patients – people like Chris Chandler, Stephen Helliar, and Stephen Britton, who have worked for decades with the communities most in need – have shown a practical path for the application of that understanding. All these role models have demonstrated what it means to be led by the communities we serve rather than trying to change them as we see fit. I don't expect to live up to these examples, but they set the standard for which to strive.

I want to acknowledge my co-workers at the West Side Community Clinic, who do incredible work each day in service of the people of Saskatoon's core neighbourhoods. I also want to recognize the board and staff at Upstream, an organization that consistently punches above its weight thanks to the new executive director, Monika Dutt, her team, Cody Sharpe, Jared Knoll, and Joanna Jakubczyk, and all the board and staff members that have contributed to its development. My thanks as well to Dean of Medicine Preston Smith, Department Head Anne Leis, and my faculty and staff colleagues in Community Health and Epidemiology at the University of Saskatchewan, especially Lisa Yeo, Erin Wolfson, Joanna Winichuk, and Carlyn Seguin in the Division of Social Accountability.

I was elected to the Saskatchewan legislature in 2017, and I am grateful to the people of Saskatoon Meewasin for allowing me to be their representative and to the incredible campaign team on that by-election and on the current leadership race. I am extremely honoured to be working alongside my NDP caucus colleagues, the caucus staff, and my constituency assistant, Jasmine Liska.

Two men of letters have had an enormous influence on my writing in general and this work in particular. Darren Dyck and Dave Mitchell are writers and editors of great talent, and I'm lucky to have them as friends. Their input has been instrumental, as has that of Olin Valby, who has a great instinct for using story to bring an idea to life.

Karen Bolstad and Don Purich took a leap of faith in publishing a first-time author and were extremely supportive in working together to make the most of this project. My thanks to them and their production team for the development of the first edition. Since the first edition, Purich Publishing has been acquired by UBC Press, and I'm thankful to the team there for all of their assistance in getting this second edition to press.

I've been thrilled to receive kind words of support from writers, thinkers, and change-makers who have influenced me. Some are close friends, others admired from afar. Names like Ashton, Barlow, Calvert, Guyatt, Marchildon, Martin, Maté, Raphael, Raza, Simard, and Yalnizyan evoke images of commitment, knowledge, and wisdom deserving of deep respect. What an honour to have them share their enthusiasm for the ideas in *A Healthy Society*.

Roy Romanow's thoughtful foreword to the first edition is a particularly high honour, as it was during the Commission on the Future of Health Care in Canada that I was inspired to join with a group of students to engage in advocacy in favour of Medicare. In subsequent years, he's become a friend and a generous contributor of advice, and it was due to his guidance that I became involved in Canadian Doctors for Medicare.

André Picard is Canada's preeminent health journalist, and his contribution of a foreword to the second edition is an exciting development. I've long been a fan of his insightful analysis of health and health care questions in Canada and am honoured to have his encouragement for this work.

Thank you for taking the time to read this book. If you think the topic is important, I hope you'll continue to read on the topic. There is no shortage of well-researched and richly described literature on the determinants of health. Because of that rich body of literature, the ideas in this book are not entirely new. The social determinants of health have found their way, in one form or another, into the works of many. Key pieces include *The Pathologies of Power* by Paul Farmer; the WHO report *Closing the Gap in a Generation: Health Equity through Action on the Social Determinants of Health*; *The Health Gap* by Michael Marmot; "Social Determinants of Health: The Canadian Facts" by Juha Mikkonen and Dennis Raphael; *Better Now* by Danielle Martin; and *Matters of Life and Death* by André Picard. This book also draws heavily on scholarly works such as the studies of Saskatoon researchers Mark Lemstra and Cory Neudorf, as well as Richard Wilkinson and Kate Pickett's *The Spirit Level*. What *A Healthy Society* does is explore these ideas in a particular context. There is some reinterpretation or reshaping, some focus on political will and the necessary conditions for change, perhaps there are even some truly new notions, and at the very least, much that bears repeating.

I would also like to invite you to take part in the conversation. Connect with organizations like Upstream at thinkupstream.net and engage politically with candidates and parties that demonstrate an understanding of the determinants of health. More importantly, it is my hope that the topic of the social determinants of health, and of a healthier body politic overall, is something you'll discuss with others. Only by engaging all citizens in the process can we have any hope of building a healthy society.

The final, and foremost, thank you goes to Mahli. I have drawn heavily on her love and support, not to mention her patience, in the preparation of this work. Sharing my life with her and our sons Abraham and Augustin is my greatest joy.

INDEX

limits and, 111–12; fiscal multipliers, 71; growth vs development, 69–70, 71–73; impacts on health, 57, 76–77; income inequality impacts, 62; laissez-faire approach, 64–65; measurements of success, 58–59, 76; minimum wage, 95–97; poverty costs, 67–69, 79; predistribution strategies, 76; profit from addressing health determinants, 67, 68; proper management for health outcomes, 65–67, 73–74; Saskatoon housing boom impact on poor, 62, 63–64; state-involved approach, 65; taxation policy, 74–76. *See also* basic income guarantee; income

Ecuador: Cotacachi, 165–66

education: affordability and accessibility issues, 133, 135–36, 141; Amy and Mason's story, 131–32, 141–42; child care, 139; civic education, 137; community schools (School Plus), 139–40; on First Nations reserves, 133–34; health education, 136–37; impacts on health, 132–33; medical school, 85–86; need to value teachers, 138; politics and, 137–38; post-secondary education, 134–35, 140–41; public investments in, 135–36; purpose of, 136–37

Elaine (housing story), 98–100

End Stage of Poverty, 6

environment: agriculture, 114–15; carbon pricing, 117–19; climate change in Western Canada, 112; climate refugees in Canada, 115–16; economic planning and, 111–12; greenhouse gases in Canada, 115, 117; impacts on health, 111, 112; Janiuay, Philippines, 110–11; political leadership needed, 116–17; poverty and climate change, 111, 116; renewable energy, 115; telling better stories about, 119–20; União, Brazil, 113–14

epidemiology, 33, 87

equity, 19, 34–35

evidence-based medicine: in Canadian Doctors for Medicare, 50; explanation of, 28; policy creation and, 28; steps for, 29–32

Falvo, Nick, 71

FIFE (feelings, ideas, functions, and expectations) interview, 25–26

Finland, 33–34

First Nations. *See* Indigenous peoples

First Nations Child and Family Caring Society of Canada, 168

fiscal multipliers, 71

food insecurity: in Canada, 101–2, 107; community-based initiatives against, 107–8; corporate and government responsibilities, 108; costs, 107; Don Bouvier's story, 100–1; housing and, 107; impacts on health, 107; income and, 108–9; pricing disparities, 108

Forget, Evelyn, 92

frames, 9–10

Francescutti, Louis, 190

freedom, 174–75

Gandhi, 176

gangs, 121–22

GDP (Gross Domestic Product), 58–59

Genuine Progress Index, 59

GIS (Guaranteed Income Supplement), 41, 109

"Global Change and Public Health" (CPHA), 112

Good Food Box, 108

Good Food Junction, 12, 187

Gottlieb, Laura, 45

Grande, David, 172

Green Economy Network, 118

greenhouse gases, 115, 117. *See also* carbon pricing

Gross Domestic Product (GDP), 58–59

Gross National Product, 58–59

Guaranteed Income Supplement (GIS), 41, 109

Guyatt, Gordon, 28

Haggie, John, 190
Halligan, Aidan, 46
Hamilton (ON), 16
Hancock, Trevor, 112
Harper, Stephen, 74, 198*n*27
HEAL ("Health Equity Action Lens") approach, 34–35
health: common preoccupation with, 10; human right to, 24; World Health Organization definition of, 18, 66. *See also* social determinants of health
health care: accessibility, 146–47; approach to, 146, 156, 158–59; costs, 149–50, 151, 157; evidence-based medicine, 28–29, 29–33; financial system, 148–49; Health Council, 155–56; impacts on health, 14, 145; innovations, 154–55, 157–58; Lynn Peters' story, 143–45; meaningful outcomes, 26; measurement of health outcomes, 145–46; Medicare, 17, 50–51, 146, 150, 156, 158; patient-centred medicine, 25–27; in politics, 10–11, 23, 183; prescription drugs Crown corporation approach, 152–54; prescription drugs universal coverage, 151–52; primary health care teams, 149; private health care system, 49, 50–51, 150, 189; public funding, 149–50, 150–51; redistribution and, 156; social accountability, 27–28, 42, 147–48; social determinants of health and, 24–25, 158; super users and medical hot spots, 157–58; sustainability of, 149–50; weakening of national system, 155–56
health care providers: advocacy role, 39, 42–43, 52; collaborative approach, 26–27; daily experience for, 13; fostering relationship with patients, 38; gifts from pharmaceutical companies, 172–73
Health Council of Canada, 155–56
health education, 136–37
"Health Equity Action Lens" (HEAL) approach, 34–35

Health in All Policies, 33–34, 185
Health Providers against Poverty, 41
heart attacks, 144
Heath, Joseph, 59
HIV/AIDS, 3, 4, 56, 82
homelessness, 63, 103–4, 104–5, 106
Hoskins, Eric, 92
housing: 1 percent solution, 103; advocacy for, 103; affordability issues, 99, 102–3, 105, 139; food insecurity and, 107; homelessness strategies for, 103–4; Housing First initiatives for homeless, 106; Jessica and Elaine's story, 98–100; lack of government investment, 102, 105; private sector involvement, 102; public investment benefits, 106–7
Housing First model, 106
Hub and Centre of Responsibility (COR) approach, 128, 157

Iceland, 129
Idle No More, 188
IFH (Interim Federal Health) program, 47–49
Île-à-la-Crosse (SK), 139–40
incarceration. *See* justice system
income: basic income guarantee, 91–95; Brazilian inequality, 113; Canadian inequality, 64; diabetes mellitus example, 60–61; economic damage from inequality, 62; food insecurity and, 108–9; importance and impacts, 55–56, 57, 79; life expectancy and, 61–62; redistribution, 61, 70, 75–76; Tevele, Mozambique example, 56–57. *See also* basic income guarantee; economy/economics
income tax. *See* taxes
Indian Posse, 121–22
Indigenous peoples: child poverty and services discrimination, 168–69; education on reserves, 133–34; health outcomes, 166–67; homelessness rates, 104; Idle No More, 188; Jordan's Principle, 168; in justice system, 123,

127–28; lack of services on reserves, 168; Truth and Reconciliation Commission, 167; voter registration, 164; working together with, 167, 169

individuality, 21

Interim Federal Health (IFH) program, 47–49

International Monetary Fund, 75

Janiuay, Philippines, 110–11

Jessica (housing story), 98–100

Jordan's Principle, 168

justice system: alternative programs and approaches, 128–29; Brad Peequaquat's story, 121–22, 129–30; costs, 126; Hub and Centre of Responsibility (COR) approach, 128, 157; Indigenous peoples in, 123, 127–28; loss of rehabilitation opportunities, 124; negative impacts from, 124–25; parallels to social determinants of health, 123, 130; profile of incarcerated youth in Saskatchewan, 127–28; reasons for punishment, 123–24; recidivism (reoffending) rates, 126–27; retribution focus, 124, 125

J.W. McConnell Family Foundation, 93

Kennedy, Bobby, 58

Kenney, Jason, 48

Kent, Steve, 185

Kershaw, Paul, 139

Kierans, Eric, 65

Kingston (ON), 124

Klass, Perri, 89

Koostachin, Shannen, 134

laissez-faire economics, 64–65

Lakoff, George, 9

Lancet, 117

laryngeal mask airway, 144

life expectancy, 61–62

Lipitor, 151

Lisa (poverty story), 80–84

living wage, 76, 96

Living Wage YXE, 96

Lloyd, Woodrow, 136

locum tenens, 143

Making the Links, 148

Manchanda, Rishi, 45–46

Manitoba, 167–68

Mann, Horace, 133

Marmot, Michael, 25, 32, 34, 43, 51, 189–90

Martin, Danielle, 49

Mason (education story), 131–32, 141

Maxine (social determinants of health story), 3–6, 21

Mazzucato, Mariana, 75

meaningful outcomes, 26

medical hot spots, 157

Medicare, 17, 50–51, 146, 150, 156, 158

medicine. *See* health care; health care providers

Medicine Hat (AB), 106

Meili, Ryan: political involvement, 183–86; political position, 176–77

Meili, Wally, 177–78

methylphenidate (Ritalin), 99

Mikkonen, Juha, 182

Mincome, 91–92

minimum wage, 76, 95–96

morality, 9

Morgan, Steve, 151

mosquito bed-nets, 161–63

Movimento Sem Terra, 114

Mozambique, 54–57, 101, 110, 113, 161–63

National Shelter Study, 104

Nenshi, Naheed, 180

neoliberalism, 64–65

Neudorf, Cory, 16

New Deal for People, 170

New Democratic Party (federal), 185

New Democratic Party (SK), 170, 184, 185

Newfoundland and Labrador, 75, 89–90, 108, 185

Nunavut, 108

nurses. *See* health care providers

Raphael, Dennis, 55–56, 182, 189, 191
Raworth, Kate, 111
recidivism (reoffending), 126–27
redistribution, wealth, 61, 70, 75–76, 156
refugee care, 47–49
Regina (SK), 106
Regina Correctional Centre, 124
Reid, Anna, 190
Remai, Joe, 187
renewable energy, 115
reoffending (recidivism), 126–27
Ritalin (methylphenidate), 99
Romanow, Roy, 150, 170
RxFiles, 28

Saskatchewan: 2011 federal election, 178–79; boom-bust cycles, 70–71, 72; child care, 139; climate refugees in, 115–16; community schools (School Plus), 139–40; equality reputation, 17; food cost disparities, 108; greenhouse gases, 115, 117; hypothetical pharmaceutical Crown corporation, 153–54; income inequality in, 62, 64; Indigenous child poverty rate, 168; political donations, 173; post-secondary tuition rates, 135; poverty reduction strategy, 90–91; prison population, 123; production-consumption loop, 73; provincial politics, 184; youth incarceration, 127–28
Saskatchewan Human Rights Commission, 137
Saskatchewan New Democratic Party, 170, 184, 185
Saskatchewan Party, 117, 164, 170, 184
Saskatoon: diabetes mellitus in, 60; downtown neighbourhoods, 11–12; food security initiatives, 107–8; health and social disparities study, 15–17, 29–31; health services super users, 157; HIV/AIDS, 82; homelessness, 104; housing boom impact on poor, 62, 63–64; St. Mary's School,

140; Station 20 West, 12–13, 157, 186–88; survey on social determinants of health, 188–89; SWITCH (Student Wellness Initiative Toward Community Health), 26–27, 46–47, 60, 148, 157
Saskatoon Housing Initiatives Partnership, 104
Saskatoon Meewasin, 184
Saskatoon Poverty Reduction Partnership, 30–31
School Plus (community schools), 139–40
Senate of Canada: *A Healthy, Productive Canada,* 160
seniors, 41, 109
Shannen's Dream, 134
shelter. *See* housing
Sick Kids Hospital (Toronto), 48
Siddall, Evan, 105
Simpson, Chris, 190
Sinclair, Murray, 167
Skinner, Stu, 6
social accountability, 27–28, 42, 147–48
social assistance, 19, 68, 76, 88, 91, 108
social determinants of health: acceptance in mainstream medicine, 24–25; advocacy for, 51–52; approach to, 21–22, 183; Canadian Medical Association's focus on, 189–90; in Canadian politics, 185–86; economic benefits of addressing, 67–69; equity approach, 19; impacts on health, 13, 15, 18; individual choice and, 21; inequality impacts, 7, 20–21; Maxine's story, 3–6; measurement frameworks for, 31–33; need for dissemination, 191; overview, 14; in Phantom Zone, 189, 190–91; political action needed for, 14–15; as political frame, 174, 182–83; Saskatoon survey on, 188–89; screening tools for, 41–42; as societal yardstick, 35; studies on, 15–17, 24–25, 29. *See also* economy/economics; education; environment; food insecurity; health care;

ABOUT THE AUTHOR

RYAN MEILI is a family physician, an upstream thinker, and the MLA for Saskatoon Meewasin. Dr. Meili has founded numerous organizations and initiatives, including Upstream: Institute for a Healthy Society, which promotes the idea that we can create a healthy society through evidence-based, people-centred policies; the Division of Social Accountability at the College of Medicine, University of Saskatchewan, which helps to ensure that Saskatchewan's future doctors are equipped to meet the needs of the diverse communities they serve; SWITCH, the Student Wellness Initiative Toward Community Health, a student-run clinic; and the College of Medicine's Making the Links program, which gives medical students the opportunity to work in Northern Saskatchewan, SWITCH, and communities in the Global South.

Dr. Meili's work has been recognized with numerous awards and honours, including the Saskatchewan College of Family Physicians Award of Excellence (2014), University of Saskatchewan Alumni Achievement Award (2015), and College of Physicians and Surgeons of Saskatchewan Distinguished Service Award (2015).

Printed and bound in Canada by Marquis

Set in Calibri and Sabon by Artegraphica Design Co. Ltd.

Copy editor: Deborah Kerr

Proofreader: Carmen Tiampo

Indexer: Stephen Ullstrom